Bariatric Meal Prep Cookbook

Delicious, Mouthwatering Recipes with Meal Planning Guides and Expert Tips for Long-Term Success

By

Dr. Janice E. Simon

Table of Contents

Welcome to the "Bariatric Meal Prep Cookbook: Delicious, Mouthwatering Recipes with Meal Planning Guides and Expert Tips for Long-Term Success." This eBook is designed to be your go-to resource for creating satisfying, nutritious meals tailored specifically to support your health journey post-bariatric surgery.

Deciding to undergo bariatric surgery is a significant step towards improving your health and well-being. However, the journey doesn't end in the operating room. Establishing sustainable habits that will support your long-term success and help you achieve and maintain your health goals is essential.

One of the cornerstones of post-bariatric success is proper nutrition. Following surgery, your body's dietary needs change, and it's crucial to adapt your eating habits accordingly. This cookbook is here to guide you through that process, providing delicious recipes, practical meal-planning guides, and expert tips to support your journey every step of the way.

Each recipe in this cookbook has been carefully crafted to provide the nutrients your body needs while satisfying your taste buds. From hearty breakfasts to flavorful dinners and everything in between, these recipes are designed to make healthy eating enjoyable and accessible.

In addition to recipes, you'll find invaluable meal-planning guides to help you stay organized and on track with your nutritional goals. We understand that life can be busy, but with proper planning and preparation, you can ensure that healthy eating fits seamlessly into your lifestyle.

Finally, we've included expert tips from professionals who understand the unique challenges and opportunities of post-bariatric living. Whether seeking advice on managing cravings, navigating social situations, or maintaining motivation, you'll find practical strategies to support your long-term success.

Thank you for choosing the "Bariatric Meal Prep Cookbook" to accompany you on your health journey. We're excited to be a part of your success and to help you discover the joy of nourishing your body with delicious, nutritious meals.

Meal Planning Guides

Meal planning is essential to maintaining a healthy and balanced diet, especially after undergoing bariatric surgery. Proper meal planning can help you stay on track with your nutritional goals, manage portion sizes, and make healthy eating more convenient and accessible. Here are some meal planning guides to help you navigate your post-bariatric journey:

Weekly Meal Planner: Start by creating a weekly meal plan outlining your daily meals. Consider your schedule, dietary preferences, and nutritional needs when planning your meals. A structured meal plan can help you stay organized and avoid last-minute unhealthy food choices.

Portion Control: After bariatric surgery, paying attention to portion sizes is essential to avoid overeating and ensure adequate nutrition. Use portion control tools such as measuring cups, food scales, or visual references (like using your hand as a guide) to help you accurately portion your meals.

Balanced Nutrients: To support your body's nutritional needs, focus on incorporating a balance of macronutrients (carbohydrates, proteins, and fats) into each meal. Aim to include lean proteins, healthy fats, complex carbohydrates, and plenty of fruits and vegetables to promote satiety and overall well-being.

Meal Prep: Spend time prepping and batch-cooking meals and snacks each week to save time and make healthy eating more convenient. Prepare larger quantities of staple ingredients such as grilled chicken, quinoa, or roasted vegetables that can be incorporated into multiple meals throughout the week.

Variety and Flexibility: Incorporate a variety of flavors, textures, and cuisines into your meal plan to keep your meals interesting and enjoyable. Don't be afraid to experiment with new recipes and ingredients to keep things fresh and exciting. Additionally, allow flexibility in your meal plan to accommodate changes in your schedule or unexpected cravings.

Hydration: Drink plenty of water and other calorie-free beverages throughout the day. Dehydration can contribute to feelings of hunger and fatigue, so aim to consume at least 64 ounces of fluids per day, or as your healthcare provider recommends.

Listen to Your Body:
1. Pay attention to your body's hunger and fullness cues, and eat mindfully without distractions.
2. Eat slowly, thoroughly chew your food, and stop eating when you feel satisfied.

3. Avoid eating past the point of fullness, as this can lead to discomfort and digestive issues.

By following these meal planning guides, you can set yourself up for success on your post-bariatric journey and make healthy eating a sustainable and enjoyable part of your lifestyle. Remember to consult your healthcare provider or a registered dietitian for personalized guidance and recommendations based on your needs and goals.

Expert Tips for Long-Term Success:

Navigating the post-bariatric journey requires more than just following a set of dietary guidelines. It involves adopting sustainable habits, addressing challenges, and embracing a holistic approach to health and well-being. Here are some expert tips to support your long-term success after bariatric surgery:

Prioritize Protein: Protein is essential for maintaining muscle mass, promoting satiety, and supporting healing after surgery. Make protein a focal point of your meals by incorporating lean sources such as poultry, fish, tofu, eggs, and legumes. Aim to include protein in every meal to help you feel full and satisfied.

Mindful Eating:

1. Practice mindful eating by paying attention to your body's hunger and fullness cues and the sensory experience of eating.
2. Slow down, chew your food thoroughly, and savor each bite.
3. Avoid distractions such as screens or multitasking while eating, as this can lead to overeating.

Stay Hydrated: Adequate hydration is crucial for overall health and digestion, especially after bariatric surgery. Aim to drink plenty of water throughout the day and prioritize fluids over sugary or calorie-laden beverages. Carry a water bottle with you as a reminder to stay hydrated and sip fluids consistently throughout the day.

Build a Support Network: Surround yourself with a supportive network of friends, family, healthcare professionals, and fellow bariatric patients who understand and empathize with your journey. Join online and in-person support groups to connect with others who can offer encouragement, advice, and camaraderie.

Physical Activity:

1. Incorporate regular physical activity into your routine to support weight loss, improve cardiovascular health, and enhance overall well-being.
2. Choose activities that you enjoy and that fit your fitness level, whether it's walking, swimming, yoga, or strength training.
3. Aim for at least 30 minutes of moderate-intensity exercise most days of the week or as recommended by your healthcare provider.

Practice Self-Compassion: Be kind to yourself and practice self-compassion as you navigate the ups and downs of your post-bariatric journey. Celebrate your successes, no matter how small, and be patient with yourself during setbacks or challenges. Remember that progress is not always linear, and asking for help when needed is okay.

Mindset Shift:
1. Shift your focus from short-term weight loss goals to long-term health and well-being.
2. Instead of viewing food as a reward or punishment, see it as nourishment for your body and fuel for your activities.
3. Cultivate a positive mindset towards food, exercise, and self-care, and embrace a lifestyle that supports your overall health and happiness.

By incorporating these expert tips into your post-bariatric lifestyle, you can set yourself up for long-term success and enjoy a fulfilling and healthy life beyond surgery. Remember that every journey is unique, so listen to your body, trust your instincts, and seek support when needed. You can achieve and maintain your health goals for years with dedication, perseverance, and a positive attitude.

Maintaining long-term success after bariatric surgery involves more than just following a strict diet or exercise regimen; it requires adopting sustainable lifestyle habits that promote overall health and well-being. Here are some strategies to help you sustain your progress and thrive on your post-bariatric journey:

Focus on Whole Foods: Emphasize whole, nutrient-dense foods such as fruits, vegetables, lean proteins, whole grains, and healthy fats. These foods provide essential vitamins, minerals, and antioxidants while promoting satiety and overall health. Limit processed and refined foods high in calories, sugar, and unhealthy fats.

Meal Prep and Planning: Set aside time each week to plan and prepare your meals in advance. Batch cooking and meal prepping can save time, reduce stress, and make healthy eating more convenient throughout the week. Invest in quality storage containers, portion control tools, and meal planning resources to streamline the process and stay organized.

Practice Portion Control:
1. Pay attention to portion sizes and avoid overeating using smaller plates, bowls, and utensils.
2. Be mindful of serving sizes and listen to your body's hunger and fullness cues to avoid excess calorie intake.
3. Avoid mindless eating in front of the TV or computer, and savor each bite by eating slowly and mindfully.

Stay Active:
1. Regular physical activity in your daily routine supports weight management, improves cardiovascular health, and enhances overall well-being.
2. Find activities that you enjoy and that fit your lifestyle, whether it's walking, biking, swimming, or dancing.
3. Aim for at least 150 minutes of moderate-intensity exercise per week, or as your healthcare provider recommends.

Build a Support System:
1. Surround yourself with a supportive network of friends, family, healthcare professionals, and fellow bariatric patients who understand and empathize with your journey.

2. Join online and in-person support groups to connect with others who can offer encouragement, advice, and accountability.
3. Share your successes, challenges, and goals with your support system and celebrate your progress.

Practice Mindful Eating:

1. Be present and mindful during meals by paying attention to the sensory experience of eating, including taste, texture, and aroma.
2. Chew your food thoroughly, eat slowly, and savor each bite.
3. Avoid distractions such as screens or multitasking while eating, and focus on enjoying your meals' nourishing and satisfying qualities.

Set Realistic Goals:

1. Set realistic and achievable goals for yourself, both short-term and long-term.
2. Break larger goals into smaller, manageable steps, and celebrate your progress.
3. Be flexible and adaptable, and recognize that setbacks are a normal part of the journey.
4. Learn from your experiences, adjust your strategies as needed, and stay committed to your health and well-being.

By implementing these sustainability strategies into your post-bariatric lifestyle, you can create lasting habits that support your overall health, happiness, and long-term success. Remember that every journey is unique, so find what works best for you and prioritize self-care, consistency, and balance in all aspects of your life. With dedication, perseverance, and a positive mindset, you can thrive on your post-bariatric journey and enjoy a fulfilling and healthy life for years.

Protein-Packed Breakfast Burrito

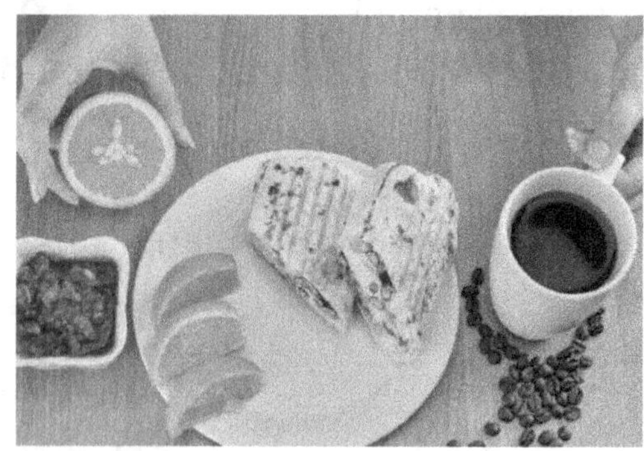

Cooking Time: 15 minutes
 Serving: 2
Materials:
- Four large eggs
- 1/4 cup diced bell peppers (any color)
- 1/4 cup diced onions
- 1/4 cup diced tomatoes
- 1/4 cup cooked black beans
- 1/4 cup diced cooked turkey sausage or bacon (optional)
- 1/4 cup shredded cheese (cheddar or Monterey Jack)
- Two large whole-wheat tortillas
- Salt and pepper to taste
- Salsa, avocado, or Greek yogurt for serving (optional)

Steps:
1. Heat a non-stick skillet over medium heat and lightly coat it with cooking spray or oil.
2. In a bowl, whisk together the eggs until well beaten. Season with salt and pepper.
3. Pour the beaten eggs into the skillet and let them cook for a minute until they start to set around the edges.
4. Add diced bell peppers, onions, and tomatoes to the skillet. Stir gently to combine with the eggs.

5. Once the eggs are mostly set but still slightly runny, add the cooked black beans and diced turkey sausage or bacon. Continue cooking, stirring occasionally, until the eggs are fully cooked and everything is heated through.
6. Sprinkle shredded cheese evenly over the egg mixture. Let it melt slightly.
7. Warm the tortillas in a separate skillet or microwave until soft and pliable.
8. Divide the egg mixture evenly between the two tortillas, placing it in each center.
9. Fold the sides of the tortillas over the filling, then roll them up tightly to form burritos.
10. Serve immediately with salsa, avocado slices, or Greek yogurt if desired.

Nutrition Facts (per serving):
- Calories: 320
- Total Fat: 15g
  - Saturated Fat: 6g
- Cholesterol: 380mg
- Sodium: 600mg
- Total Carbohydrates: 25g
  - Dietary Fiber: 5g
  - Sugars: 3g
- Protein: 21g

Spinach and Feta Egg Muffins

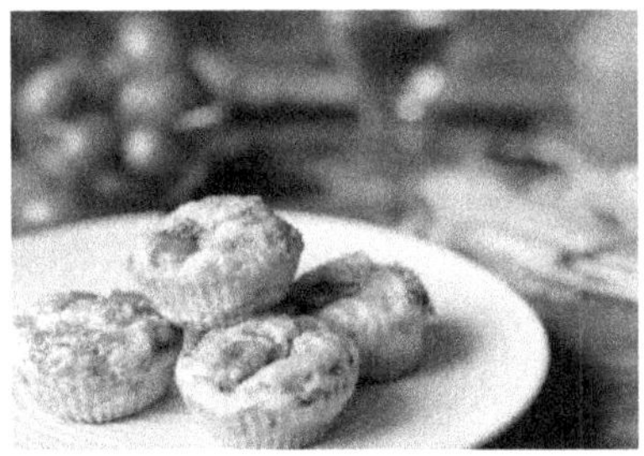

Cooking Time: 25 minutes
 Serving: Makes 12 muffins
Materials:
- Eight large eggs
- 1 cup fresh spinach, chopped
- 1/2 cup crumbled feta cheese

- 1/4 cup milk
- 1/4 teaspoon salt
- 1/4 teaspoon black pepper
- Cooking spray or olive oil for greasing muffin tin

Steps:

1. Preheat your oven to 350°F (175°C). Grease a 12-cup muffin tin with cooking spray or olive oil.
2. In a large mixing bowl, crack the eggs and beat them well.
3. Add chopped spinach, crumbled feta cheese, milk, salt, and black pepper to the beaten eggs. Mix until all ingredients are well combined.
4. Pour the egg mixture evenly into each muffin cup, filling them about 3/4 full.
5. Place the muffin tin in the preheated oven and bake for 20-25 minutes until the muffins are set and the tops are lightly golden.
6. Once done, remove the muffin tin from the oven and allow the muffins to cool for a few minutes.
7. Use a knife or spatula to gently loosen the edges of the muffins, then transfer them to a wire rack to cool completely.
8. Serve the spinach and feta egg muffins warm or at room temperature. Enjoy!

Nutrition Facts:

- Serving Size: 1 muffin
- Calories: 90
- Total Fat: 6g
    - Saturated Fat: 2g
    - Trans Fat: 0g
- Cholesterol: 150mg
- Sodium: 180mg
- Total Carbohydrates: 1g
    - Dietary Fiber: 0g
    - Sugars: 0g
- Protein: 7g

Greek Yogurt Parfait with Berries

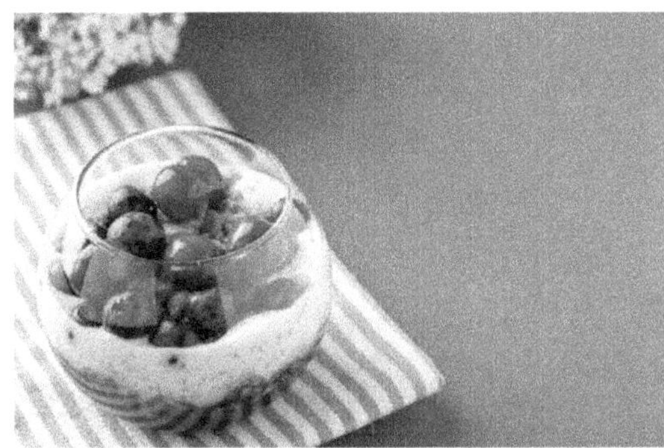

Cooking Time: 10 minutes
 Servings: 2
Materials:
- 1 cup Greek yogurt
- 1 cup mixed berries (strawberries, blueberries, raspberries)
- Two tablespoons of honey or maple syrup
- 1/4 cup granola
- Fresh mint leaves for garnish (optional)

Steps:
1. **Prepare the Berries:** Wash the berries thoroughly under cold water and pat them dry with a paper towel. If using strawberries, hull and slice them.
2. **Layering the Parfait:** Spoon a layer of Greek yogurt into the bottom of two serving glasses or bowls.
3. **Add Berries:** Add a layer of mixed berries on top of the yogurt.
4. **Drizzle with Sweetener:** Drizzle honey or maple syrup over the berries for added sweetness.
5. **Repeat Layers:** Repeat the layers until the glasses are filled, alternating between yogurt, berries, and sweetener.
6. **Top with Granola:** Sprinkle granola evenly over the top of each parfait.
7. **Garnish:** Garnish with fresh mint leaves for added freshness and presentation if desired.
8. **Serve:** Serve immediately or refrigerate until ready to serve.

Nutrition Facts (per serving):
- Calories: 200
- Total Fat: 5g
- Saturated Fat: 1g

- Cholesterol: 10mg
- Sodium: 50mg
- Total Carbohydrates: 30g
- Dietary Fiber: 5g
- Sugars: 20g
- Protein: 15g

Cottage Cheese Pancakes

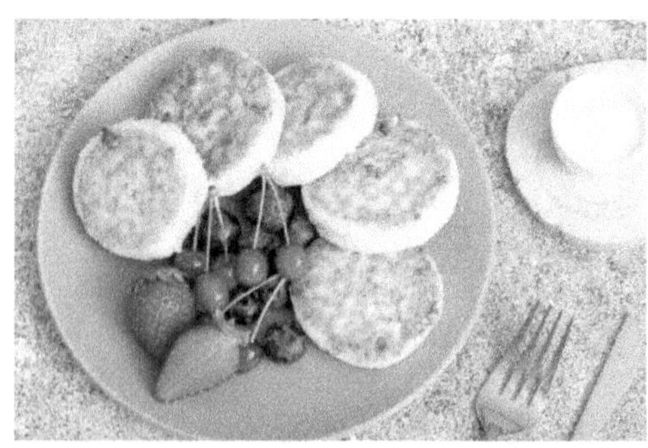

Cooking Time: 15 minutes
Serving: 4
Materials:
- 1 cup cottage cheese
- Four eggs
- 1/4 cup all-purpose flour
- Two tablespoons sugar
- One teaspoon of vanilla extract
- 1/4 teaspoon salt
- Butter or oil for frying
- Optional toppings: fresh fruit, maple syrup, honey, or powdered sugar

Steps:
1. Combine cottage cheese, eggs, flour, sugar, vanilla extract, and salt in a mixing bowl. Mix until well combined and smooth batter forms.
2. Heat a skillet or frying pan over medium heat and add a small amount of butter or oil to grease the surface.
3. Spoon about 1/4 cup of batter onto the skillet for each pancake. Cook for 2-3 minutes on each side until golden brown is cooked through.
4. Repeat with the remaining batter, adding more butter or oil to the skillet as needed.

5. Serve the pancakes warm with your choice of toppings, such as fresh fruit, maple syrup, honey, or powdered sugar.

Nutrition Facts (per serving):
- Calories: 220
- Total Fat: 10g
    - Saturated Fat: 4g
    - Trans Fat: 0g
- Cholesterol: 200mg
- Sodium: 360mg
- Total Carbohydrate: 16g
    - Dietary Fiber: 1g
    - Sugars: 6g
- Protein: 15g
- Vitamin D: 10%
- Calcium: 10%
- Iron: 6%
- Potassium: 4%

Veggie Omelet Roll-Ups

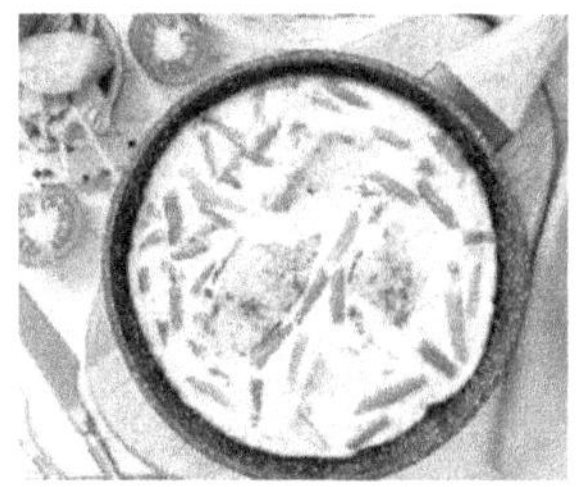

Cooking Time: 15 minutes
 Servings: 2
Materials:
- Four large eggs
- 1/4 cup diced bell peppers (any color)
- 1/4 cup diced tomatoes
- 1/4 cup chopped spinach
- Salt and pepper to taste
- One tablespoon of olive oil
- 1/4 cup shredded cheese (optional)

- Salsa or hot sauce for serving (optional)

Steps:

1. **Prepare the Ingredients:** Crack the eggs into a bowl and beat them lightly with a fork. Dice the bell peppers and tomatoes, and chop the spinach.
2. **Season the Eggs:** Season the beaten eggs with salt and pepper according to your preference.
3. **Saute the Veggies:** Heat the olive oil in a non-stick skillet over medium heat. Add the diced bell peppers and tomatoes to the skillet and sauté for 2-3 minutes until they soften. Add the chopped spinach and cook for another 1-2 minutes until wilted. Remove the veggies from the skillet and set aside.
4. **Cook the Omelet:** In the same skillet, pour the beaten eggs evenly to make a thin layer. Let the eggs cook for about 2-3 minutes until the edges start to set.
5. **Add the Veggies and Cheese:** Sprinkle the sautéed veggies evenly over the omelet. If desired, sprinkle shredded cheese on top of the veggies.
6. **Roll-Up the Omelet:** Using a spatula, gently roll up the omelet from one side to create a roll-up. Let it cook for another minute to ensure the cheese melts and the roll-up holds its shape.
7. **Slice and Serve:** Once cooked, remove the omelet roll-up from the skillet and transfer it to a cutting board. Slice the roll-up into 1-inch thick slices.
8. **Serve:** Serve the Veggie Omelet Roll-Ups hot with salsa or hot sauce on the side if desired.

Nutrition Facts (per serving):

- Calories: 180
- Total Fat: 12g
- Saturated Fat: 3.5g
- Cholesterol: 370mg
- Sodium: 220mg
- Total Carbohydrates: 5g
- Dietary Fiber: 1g
- Sugars: 2g
- Protein: 13g

Chia Seed Pudding with Almond Butter
Cooking Time: 10 minutes (plus chilling time)
 Serving: 2
Materials:

- 1/4 cup chia seeds
- 1 cup almond milk (or any milk of your choice)
- Two tablespoons of almond butter
- One tablespoon of maple syrup or honey
- 1/2 teaspoon vanilla extract
- Sliced almonds and berries for topping (optional)

Steps:

1. Combine chia seeds, almond milk, almond butter, maple syrup (or honey), and vanilla extract in a mixing bowl. Stir well to ensure everything is evenly mixed.
2. Let the mixture sit for about 5 minutes, then stir again to prevent clumping.
3. Cover the bowl with plastic wrap or a lid and refrigerate for at least 2 hours, or overnight, until the mixture thickens and resembles pudding consistency.
4. Once chilled and thickened, stir the pudding. If it's too thick, add an almond milk splash to reach your desired consistency.
5. Serve the chia seed pudding in individual bowls or jars, and top with sliced almonds and berries if desired.

Nutrition Facts (per serving):

- Calories: 220
- Total Fat: 14g
  - Saturated Fat: 1g
  - Trans Fat: 0g
- Cholesterol: 0mg
- Sodium: 90mg
- Total Carbohydrates: 20g
  - Dietary Fiber: 12g
  - Sugars: 6g
- Protein: 7g

Turkey Sausage and Vegetable Frittata

Cooking Time: 25 minutes

 Serving: 4

Materials:

- Eight large eggs
- ½ cup milk
- 1 cup diced turkey sausage
- One bell pepper, diced

- One small onion, diced
- 1 cup sliced mushrooms
- 1 cup cherry tomatoes, halved
- 1 cup baby spinach
- 1 cup shredded cheddar cheese
- Salt and pepper to taste
- Two tablespoons olive oil

Steps:

1. Preheat your oven to 350°F (175°C).
2. In a large mixing bowl, whisk eggs and milk until well combined. Season with salt and pepper to taste.
3. Heat olive oil in a large oven-safe skillet over medium heat. Add diced turkey sausage and cook until browned about 3-4 minutes.
4. Add diced bell pepper, onion, and sliced mushrooms to the skillet. Sauté until vegetables are tender, about 5 minutes.
5. Add cherry tomatoes and baby spinach to the skillet. Cook until spinach is wilted, about 2 minutes.
6. Pour the egg mixture evenly over the sausage and vegetable mixture in the skillet. Sprinkle shredded cheddar cheese on top.
7. Transfer the skillet to the preheated oven and bake for 12-15 minutes, or until the eggs are set and the cheese is melted and bubbly.
8. Remove from the oven and let it cool for a few minutes before slicing. Serve warm.

Nutrition Facts (per serving):

- Calories: 320
- Total Fat: 21g
- Saturated Fat: 8g
- Cholesterol: 400mg
- Sodium: 600mg
- Total Carbohydrate: 8g
- Dietary Fiber: 2g
- Sugars: 4g
- Protein: 25g

Avocado and Egg Breakfast Bowl
Cooking Time: 10 minutes
 Serving: 1
Materials:

- One ripe avocado

- Two eggs
- One tablespoon olive oil
- Salt and pepper to taste
- Optional toppings: diced tomatoes, sliced green onions, crumbled feta cheese, hot sauce

Steps:
1. **Prepare the Avocado:** Cut the avocado in half and remove the pit. Scoop out some avocado flesh from each half to create a larger well for the eggs.
2. **Cook the Eggs:** Heat olive oil in a skillet over medium heat. Crack the eggs into the skillet and cook until the whites are set but the yolks are still runny, for about 3-4 minutes. Season with salt and pepper.
3. **Assemble the Bowl:** Place the avocado halves on a plate or bowl. Carefully transfer one egg into each avocado half.
4. **Add Toppings:** Sprinkle your desired toppings over the eggs and avocado. Options include diced tomatoes, sliced green onions, crumbled feta cheese, or a drizzle of hot sauce.
5. **Serve:** Enjoy your Avocado and Egg Breakfast Bowl immediately while the eggs remain warm.

Nutrition Facts:
- Calories: 380
- Total Fat: 30g
- Saturated Fat: 5g
- Cholesterol: 370mg
- Sodium: 270mg
- Total Carbohydrates: 15g
- Dietary Fiber: 10g
- Sugars: 2g
- Protein: 14g

Quinoa Breakfast Porridge with Fresh Fruit
Cooking Time: 20 minutes
Serving: 2
Materials:
- 1 cup quinoa
- 2 cups water
- 1 cup milk (dairy or plant-based)
- One tablespoon honey or maple syrup
- One teaspoon vanilla extract
- Pinch of salt

- Fresh fruit of your choice (berries, sliced banana, diced apple, etc.)
- Nuts or seeds for topping (optional)

Steps:
1. Rinse the quinoa under cold water to remove any bitter coating.
2. In a saucepan, combine the rinsed quinoa and water. Bring to a boil over medium-high heat.
3. Once boiling, reduce the heat to low and cover the saucepan. Simmer for about 15 minutes until the quinoa is cooked and the water is absorbed.
4. Stir in the milk, honey or maple syrup, vanilla extract, and a pinch of salt. Cook for 5 minutes, stirring occasionally, until the mixture thickens to your desired consistency.
5. Remove the saucepan from the heat and let it cool slightly.
6. If desired, serve the quinoa porridge in bowls, topped with fresh fruit and nuts or seeds.

Nutrition Facts (per serving):
- Calories: 290
- Total Fat: 4g
- Saturated Fat: 1g
- Cholesterol: 5mg
- Sodium: 100mg
- Total Carbohydrates: 55g
- Dietary Fiber: 6g
- Sugars: 16g
- Protein: 10g

Breakfast Turkey Meatballs with Sweet Potato Hash
Cooking Time: 30 minutes
 Servings: 4
Materials:
For Turkey Meatballs:
- 1 pound ground turkey
- 1/4 cup breadcrumbs
- 1/4 cup grated Parmesan cheese
- One egg
- Two cloves garlic, minced
- One teaspoon dried thyme
- Salt and pepper to taste

For Sweet Potato Hash:
- Two large sweet potatoes, peeled and diced

- One onion, diced
- One red bell pepper, diced
- Two tablespoons olive oil
- One teaspoon paprika
- Salt and pepper to taste
- Fresh parsley, chopped (for garnish)

Steps:

1. Preheat your oven to 400°F (200°C) and line a baking sheet with parchment paper.
2. Combine ground turkey, breadcrumbs, Parmesan cheese, egg, minced garlic, dried thyme, salt, and pepper in a large bowl. Mix well until everything is evenly incorporated.
3. Form the turkey mixture into small meatballs, about 1 inch in diameter, and place them on the prepared baking sheet.
4. Bake the turkey meatballs in the oven for 15-20 minutes or until they are cooked through and golden brown.
5. While the meatballs are baking, prepare the sweet potato hash. Heat olive oil in a large skillet over medium heat. Add diced sweet potatoes, onion, and red bell pepper to the skillet. Cook, stirring occasionally, until the sweet potatoes are tender and slightly browned, about 10-12 minutes.
6. Season the sweet potato hash with paprika, salt, and pepper to taste. Stir well to combine all the flavors.
7. Once the turkey meatballs are cooked, serve them alongside the sweet potato hash. Garnish with freshly chopped parsley.

Nutrition Facts:

- Serving Size: 1/4 of the recipe
- Calories: 320
- Total Fat: 14g
- Saturated Fat: 3.5g
- Cholesterol: 125mg
- Sodium: 340mg
- Total Carbohydrates: 23g
- Dietary Fiber: 4g
- Sugars: 6g
- Protein: 25g

Zucchini and Cheese Mini Quiches
Cooking Time: 30 minutes
 Serving: Makes 12 mini quiches
Materials:
- One medium zucchini, grated
- 1 cup shredded cheese (cheddar or your choice)
- Four large eggs
- 1/2 cup milk
- Salt and pepper to taste
- 1/4 teaspoon garlic powder
- 1/4 teaspoon onion powder
- 1/4 teaspoon dried thyme
- 1/4 cup chopped fresh parsley
- Cooking spray

Steps:
1. Preheat your oven to 375°F (190°C) and lightly grease a 12-cup mini muffin tin with cooking spray.
2. In a mixing bowl, whisk the eggs, milk, salt, pepper, garlic powder, onion powder, and dried thyme until well combined.
3. Stir in the grated zucchini, shredded cheese, and chopped parsley until evenly distributed throughout the egg mixture.
4. Pour the mixture evenly into the prepared mini muffin tin, filling each cup about 3/4 full.
5. Place the muffin tin in the preheated oven and bake for 20-25 minutes until the quiches are set and lightly golden on top.
6. Once cooked, remove the mini quiches from the oven and allow them to cool in the tin for a few minutes before carefully transferring them to a wire rack to cool completely.
7. Serve warm or at room temperature, and enjoy!

Nutrition Facts (per serving):
- Calories: 97
- Total Fat: 6g
    - Saturated Fat: 3g
    - Trans Fat: 0g
- Cholesterol: 91mg
- Sodium: 134mg
- Total Carbohydrates: 3g
    - Dietary Fiber: 1g
    - Sugars: 1g

- Protein: 7g
- Vitamin D: 1mcg
- Calcium: 126mg
- Iron: 1mg
- Potassium: 120mg

Overnight Oats with Mixed Nuts and Honey
Cooking Time: 5 minutes (plus overnight chilling)
 Serving: 2
Materials:
- 1 cup rolled oats
- 1 cup milk (dairy or non-dairy)
- Two tablespoons honey
- 1/4 cup mixed nuts (such as almonds, walnuts, pecans)
- 1/2 teaspoon vanilla extract (optional)
- Pinch of salt
- Fresh fruit (optional for topping)

Steps:
1. **Prepare the Base:** In a mixing bowl, combine rolled oats, milk, honey, mixed nuts, vanilla extract (if using), and a pinch of salt. Stir until well combined.
2. **Divide into Containers:** Transfer the oat mixture into two jars or containers with lids.
3. **Chill Overnight:** Seal the jars tightly and refrigerate overnight or for at least 6-8 hours.
4. **Serve** the next morning, and give the oats a good stir. Top with fresh fruit, such as berries or sliced banana, before serving.

Nutrition Facts:
- *Serving Size:* 1/2 of the recipe
- *Calories:* Approximately 250
- *Total Fat:* 9g
- *Saturated Fat:* 1g
- *Cholesterol:* 0mg
- *Sodium:* 80mg
- *Total Carbohydrates:* 37g
- *Dietary Fiber:* 5g
- *Sugars:* 13g
- *Protein:* 7g

Bariatric-Friendly Smoothie Bowl

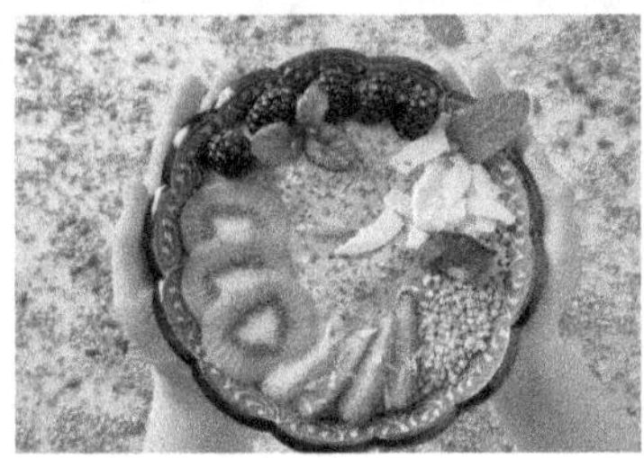

Cooking Time: 10 minutes
 Serving: 1
Materials:
- 1/2 cup frozen mixed berries
- 1/2 ripe banana, sliced and frozen
- 1/4 cup Greek yogurt (low-fat or non-fat)
- 1/4 cup unsweetened almond milk
- One tablespoon chia seeds
- One tablespoon unsweetened shredded coconut
- One tablespoon almond butter
- One teaspoon honey or maple syrup (optional, adjust to taste)
- Toppings (optional): sliced fresh fruit, nuts, seeds, granola

Steps:
1. **Prepare Ingredients:** Gather all the ingredients and ensure the banana and berries are frozen beforehand.
2. **Blend:** In a blender, combine the frozen mixed berries, frozen banana slices, Greek yogurt, almond milk, chia seeds, shredded coconut, almond butter, and honey or maple syrup. Blend until smooth and creamy.
3. **Adjust Consistency:** If the mixture is too thick, add a little more almond milk until it reaches your desired consistency.
4. **Pour and Serve:** Pour the smoothie mixture into a bowl.
5. **Add Toppings:** For added texture and flavor, top the smoothie bowl with your desired toppings, such as sliced fresh fruit, nuts, seeds, or granola.
6. **Enjoy:** Serve immediately and enjoy your delicious and nutritious bariatric-friendly smoothie bowl!

Nutrition Facts (per serving):
- Calories: 300
- Total Fat: 12g
    - Saturated Fat: 3g

- Trans Fat: 0g
- Cholesterol: 5mg
- Sodium: 80mg
- Total Carbohydrates: 40g
  - Dietary Fiber: 9g
  - Sugars: 22g
- Protein: 12g

Baked Egg Cups with Tomato and Basil
Cooking Time: 20 minutes
 Servings: 4
Materials:
- Eight large eggs
- Two medium tomatoes, diced
- 1/4 cup fresh basil leaves, chopped
- 1/2 cup shredded mozzarella cheese
- Salt and pepper to taste
- Cooking spray

Steps:
1. Preheat your oven to 375°F (190°C). Grease a muffin tin with cooking spray.
2. In a bowl, crack the eggs and whisk them together until well beaten.
3. Season the beaten eggs with salt and pepper to taste.
4. Divide the diced tomatoes and chopped basil evenly among the muffin tin cups.
5. Pour the beaten eggs over the tomatoes and basil, filling each muffin cup about 3/4 full.
6. Sprinkle shredded mozzarella cheese over the top of each egg cup.
7. Place the muffin tin in the preheated oven and bake for 15-18 minutes, until the egg is set and the cheese is melted and slightly golden on top.
8. Once baked, remove the egg cups from the oven and let them cool for a few minutes.
9. Use a spoon or knife to gently loosen the egg cups from the muffin tin, then transfer them to a serving plate.
10. Serve the baked egg cups warm, and enjoy!

Nutrition Facts (per serving):
- Calories: 180
- Total Fat: 12g
- Saturated Fat: 5g

- Cholesterol: 385mg
- Sodium: 230mg
- Total Carbohydrates: 3g
- Dietary Fiber: 1g
- Sugars: 2g
- Protein: 15g

Protein-Packed Breakfast Casserole
Cooking Time: 1 hour
 Serving: 6
Materials:
- Eight large eggs
- 1 cup cooked quinoa
- 1 cup diced cooked turkey sausage
- 1 cup chopped spinach
- 1/2 cup diced bell peppers
- 1/2 cup diced onions
- 1 cup shredded cheddar cheese
- Salt and pepper to taste
- Cooking spray or olive oil for greasing

Steps:
1. Preheat your oven to 350°F (175°C). Grease a 9x13-inch baking dish with cooking spray or olive oil.
2. In a large mixing bowl, crack the eggs and whisk them together until well beaten.
3. Add cooked quinoa, diced turkey sausage, chopped spinach, diced bell peppers, diced onions, and shredded cheddar cheese to the bowl with eggs. Mix well to combine all ingredients evenly.
4. Season the mixture with salt and pepper to taste, ensuring it is well seasoned.
5. Pour the mixture into the prepared baking dish, spreading it out evenly.
6. Place the baking dish in the oven and bake for 35-40 minutes until the eggs are set and the top is golden brown.
7. Once cooked, remove the casserole from the oven and let it cool for a few minutes before slicing and serving.
8. Serve the protein-packed breakfast casserole warm, either on its own or with fresh fruit or avocado slices.

Nutrition Facts (per serving):
- Calories: 290

- Total Fat: 17g
    - Saturated Fat: 7g
- Cholesterol: 310mg
- Sodium: 420mg
- Total Carbohydrates: 12g
    - Dietary Fiber: 2g
    - Sugars: 2g
- Protein: 21g

Cottage Cheese and Berry Stuffed Crepes
Cooking Time: 30 minutes
 Serving: Makes six crepes
Materials:
- For the Crepes:
    - 1 cup all-purpose flour
    - 1 1/2 cups milk
    - Two large eggs
    - Two tablespoons melted butter
    - Pinch of salt
- For the Filling:
    - 1 cup cottage cheese
    - 1 cup mixed berries (strawberries, blueberries, raspberries)
    - Two tablespoons honey
    - One teaspoon vanilla extract
- Additional:
    - Butter or cooking spray for greasing the pan
    - Powdered sugar for dusting (optional)

Steps:
1. **Prepare the Crepe Batter:**
    - In a mixing bowl, whisk together flour and salt.
    - In another bowl, whisk together milk, eggs, and melted butter.
    - Gradually pour the wet ingredients into the dry ingredients, whisking continuously until smooth batter forms. Let it rest for 10 minutes.
1. **Cook the Crepes:**
    - Heat a non-stick skillet over medium heat and lightly grease it with butter or cooking spray.
    - Pour 1/4 cup of the batter into the skillet and swirl it around to form a thin, even layer.

- Cook the crepe for 2 minutes until the edges lift and the bottom is lightly golden. Flip and cook for another minute on the other side.
- Repeat with the remaining batter. Stack the cooked crepes on a plate and cover with a clean kitchen towel to keep warm.

1. **Prepare the Filling:**
   - Combine cottage cheese, mixed berries, honey, and vanilla extract in a mixing bowl. Mix well until evenly combined.
1. **Assemble the Crepes:**
   - Spoon a generous portion of the cottage cheese and berry filling onto each crepe.
   - Roll up the crepes and place them seam-side down on a serving plate.
1. **Serve:**
   - Dust the stuffed crepes with powdered sugar, if desired.
   - Serve warm and enjoy!

Nutrition Facts (per serving):
- Calories: 240
- Total Fat: 9g
- Saturated Fat: 5g
- Cholesterol: 95mg
- Sodium: 230mg
- Total Carbohydrate: 30g
- Dietary Fiber: 2g
- Sugars: 11g
- Protein: 10g

Southwest Breakfast Bowl with Black Beans and Avocado
Cooking Time: 15 minutes
 Serving: 2
Materials:
- 1 cup cooked quinoa
- 1 cup black beans, cooked and drained
- One ripe avocado, sliced
- 1 cup cherry tomatoes, halved
- 1/2 cup corn kernels, cooked
- 1/4 cup red onion, finely chopped
- 1/4 cup cilantro, chopped
- One lime, juiced
- Two eggs, cooked to preference (fried, poached, or scrambled)

- Salt and pepper to taste
- Optional toppings: salsa, hot sauce, shredded cheese

Steps:

1. **Prepare Ingredients:** Cook the quinoa according to the package instructions. Rinse and drain the black beans. Slice the avocado and cherry tomatoes. If the corn kernels are not already cooked, cook them. Finely chop the red onion and cilantro. Juice the lime.
2. **Assemble the Bowl:** Divide cooked quinoa between two serving bowls. Top each bowl with half of the black beans, avocado slices, cherry tomatoes, corn kernels, red onion, and cilantro.
3. **Season:** Drizzle lime juice over each bowl. Season with salt and pepper to taste.
4. **Add Eggs:** Place a cooked egg on top of each bowl.
5. **Optional Toppings:** If desired, garnish with salsa, hot sauce, or shredded cheese.
6. **Serve:** Serve immediately and enjoy a delicious and nutritious Southwest breakfast bowl!

Nutrition Facts (per serving):

- Calories: 420
- Total Fat: 19g
    - Saturated Fat: 3g
    - Trans Fat: 0g
- Cholesterol: 186mg
- Sodium: 125mg
- Total Carbohydrates: 49g
    - Dietary Fiber: 14g
    - Sugars: 4g
- Protein: 18g

Bariatric-Friendly Breakfast Sandwich with Turkey Bacon
Cooking Time: 15 minutes
Servings: 1
Materials:

- Two slices whole grain sandwich bread (choose a brand with lower carb and higher fiber content)
- Two slices turkey bacon
- One large egg
- One slice of reduced-fat cheese (such as cheddar or Swiss)
- Non-stick cooking spray

- Salt and pepper to taste
- Optional: sliced avocado, tomato, or spinach for extra nutrients

Steps:

1. **Prepare the Ingredients:** Heat a non-stick skillet over medium heat. While the skillet heats up, toast the two slices of whole-grain bread until lightly browned. Set aside. Cook the turkey bacon according to package instructions until crispy. Remove from skillet and set aside.
2. **Cook the Egg:** Spray the skillet with non-stick cooking spray. Crack the egg into the skillet and season with salt and pepper to taste. Cook until the egg white is set and the yolk reaches your desired consistency (typically about 2-3 minutes for a runny yolk). Flip the egg if desired for even cooking.
3. **Assemble the Sandwich:** Place one slice of the toasted bread on a plate. Top with the cooked turkey bacon, followed by the cooked egg. Add the slice of reduced-fat cheese on top of the egg. If desired, add any optional toppings, such as sliced avocado, tomato, or spinach.
4. **Top and Serve:** Place the second slice of toasted bread on the cheese to complete the sandwich. Press down gently to help the ingredients stick together. Serve immediately while warm.

Nutrition Facts:

- **Calories:** Approximately 300-350 (depending on bread and additional toppings)
- **Protein:** Approximately 20-25 grams
- **Carbohydrates:** Approximately 25-30 grams (depending on bread and additional toppings)
- **Fat:** Approximately 15-20 grams (depending on the type of cheese and bacon)
- **Fiber:** Approximately 5-8 grams (depending on bread and additional toppings)

Cauliflower Hash Browns

Cooking Time: 30 minutes

 Servings: 4

Materials:

- One medium head of cauliflower
- One egg
- 1/4 cup grated Parmesan cheese
- 1/4 cup breadcrumbs
- 1/2 teaspoon garlic powder

- 1/2 teaspoon onion powder
- Salt and pepper to taste
- Cooking oil (olive oil or vegetable oil)

Steps:

1. Preheat your oven to 400°F (200°C). Line a baking sheet with parchment paper or lightly grease it with cooking oil.
2. Wash the cauliflower thoroughly and remove the stem. Cut the cauliflower into florets.
3. Place the cauliflower florets in a food processor and pulse until they reach a rice-like consistency.
4. Transfer the cauliflower rice to a microwave-safe bowl and microwave on high for 4-5 minutes or until it's softened. Alternatively, steam the cauliflower rice for about 5-7 minutes.
5. Once the cauliflower rice is cooked, allow it to cool slightly, then transfer it to a clean kitchen towel or cheesecloth. Squeeze out as much excess moisture as possible.
6. Combine the squeezed cauliflower rice, egg, Parmesan cheese, breadcrumbs, garlic powder, onion powder, salt, and pepper in a mixing bowl. Mix until well combined.
7. Take a portion of the mixture and shape it into a hash brown patty. Repeat with the remaining mixture.
8. Heat a non-stick skillet over medium heat and add a drizzle of cooking oil.
9. Once the oil is hot, carefully place the cauliflower hash browns in the skillet. Cook for 3-4 minutes on each side until golden brown and crispy.
10. Transfer the cooked hash browns to the prepared baking sheet and place them in the preheated oven for 10-15 minutes to ensure they are fully cooked and crispy.
11. Once done, remove the hash browns from the oven and serve hot. This is a delicious and healthy alternative to traditional hash browns.

Nutrition Facts (per serving):

- Calories: 120
- Total Fat: 6g
- Saturated Fat: 2g
- Cholesterol: 43mg
- Sodium: 240mg
- Total Carbohydrate: 10g
- Dietary Fiber: 3g
- Sugars: 3g
- Protein: 7g

Mini Breakfast Pizzas with Turkey Sausage
Cooking Time: 20 minutes
 Servings: 4
Materials:
- 4 English muffins, split
- ½ cup pizza sauce
- 1 cup shredded mozzarella cheese
- 4 ounces cooked turkey sausage, crumbled
- Four large eggs
- Salt and pepper to taste
- Chopped fresh parsley for garnish (optional)

Steps:
1. Preheat your oven to 375°F (190°C).
2. Place the English muffin halves on a baking sheet and cut side up.
3. Spread pizza sauce evenly over each half of the English muffin.
4. Sprinkle shredded mozzarella cheese over the sauce.
5. Distribute the crumbled turkey sausage over the cheese.
6. Create a small well in the center of each pizza.
7. Crack one egg into each well. Season with salt and pepper.
8. Bake in the preheated oven for about 15-20 minutes or until the egg whites are set and the yolks are cooked to your desired consistency.
9. Remove from the oven and let cool for a few minutes.
10. Garnish with chopped parsley if desired.
11. Serve hot, and enjoy your delicious Mini Breakfast Pizzas!

Nutrition Facts:
- **Calories:** Approximately 320 per serving
- **Total Fat:** 14g
  - Saturated Fat: 6g
  - Trans Fat: 0g
- **Cholesterol:** 225mg
- **Sodium:** 710mg
- **Total Carbohydrates:** 28g
  - Dietary Fiber: 2g
  - Sugars: 3g
- **Protein:** 20g

Spinach and Mushroom Breakfast Quesadilla
Cooking Time: 20 minutes
 Serving: 2
Materials:
- Four large flour tortillas
- 1 cup sliced mushrooms
- 2 cups fresh spinach leaves
- 1 cup shredded cheddar cheese
- Four large eggs
- Salt and pepper to taste
- Two tablespoons olive oil

Steps:
1. **Prep Ingredients:** Slice mushrooms, shred cheese, and beat the eggs in a bowl. Wash spinach leaves and pat them dry.
2. **Saute Mushrooms and Spinach:** Heat 1 tablespoon of olive oil in a skillet over medium heat. Add sliced mushrooms and sauté until they release moisture and become golden brown, about 5 minutes. Add spinach leaves and cook until wilted about 2 minutes. Season with salt and pepper to taste. Remove from heat and set aside.
3. **Prepare the Quesadillas:** Place a tortilla on a flat surface. Spread a layer of shredded cheese evenly over half of the tortilla. Spoon some of the mushroom and spinach mixture over the cheese. Top with some beaten eggs. Fold the tortilla in half to cover the filling.
4. **Cook the Quesadillas:** Heat a non-stick skillet over medium heat and add 1/2 tablespoon olive oil. Carefully transfer the assembled quesadilla to the skillet and cook until golden brown and crispy on both sides, about 2-3 minutes per side. Repeat with the remaining tortillas and filling.
5. **Serve:** Once cooked, transfer the quesadillas to a cutting board and let them cool for a minute. Then, slice each quesadilla into wedges and serve hot.

Nutrition Facts (per serving):
- Calories: 420
- Total Fat: 25g
- Saturated Fat: 9g
- Cholesterol: 260mg
- Sodium: 670mg
- Total Carbohydrates: 30g
- Dietary Fiber: 3g
- Sugars: 2g

- Protein: 20g

Blueberry Almond Baked Oatmeal Cups
Cooking Time: 30 minutes
 Servings: 12 cups
Materials:
- 2 cups old-fashioned rolled oats
- 1/4 cup almond flour
- 1/4 cup sliced almonds
- One teaspoon baking powder
- 1/2 teaspoon ground cinnamon
- 1/4 teaspoon salt
- Two ripe bananas, mashed
- Two eggs
- 1/4 cup honey or maple syrup
- One teaspoon vanilla extract
- 1 cup almond milk (or any milk of your choice)
- 1 cup fresh blueberries

Steps:
1. Preheat your oven to 350°F (175°C). Grease a 12-cup muffin tin or line it with cupcake liners.
2. Combine the rolled oats, almond flour, sliced almonds, baking powder, cinnamon, and salt in a large mixing bowl.
3. Whisk together the mashed bananas, eggs, honey or maple syrup, vanilla extract, and almond milk until well combined.
4. Pour the wet ingredients into the dry ingredients and mix until just combined.
5. Gently fold in the fresh blueberries.
6. Divide the mixture evenly among the prepared muffin cups, filling each about 3/4 full.
7. Bake in the oven for 25-30 minutes or until the tops are golden brown and a toothpick inserted into the center comes clean.
8. Allow the oatmeal cups to cool in the muffin tin for a few minutes before transferring them to a wire rack to cool completely.
9. Serve warm or at room temperature. Store any leftovers in an airtight container in the refrigerator for up to 3 days.

Nutrition Facts (per serving):
- Calories: 150
- Total Fat: 5g

- Saturated Fat: 0.5g
    - Trans Fat: 0g
  - Cholesterol: 30mg
  - Sodium: 100mg
  - Total Carbohydrate: 25g
    - Dietary Fiber: 3g
    - Sugars: 10g
  - Protein: 4g

Banana Nut Protein Muffins
Cooking Time: 25 minutes
 Serving: 12 muffins
Materials:
- Two ripe bananas
- Two eggs
- 1/4 cup honey or maple syrup
- 1/4 cup unsweetened applesauce
- 1/4 cup Greek yogurt
- One teaspoon vanilla extract
- 1 1/2 cups almond flour
- 1/4 cup vanilla protein powder
- One teaspoon baking powder
- 1/2 teaspoon baking soda
- 1/4 teaspoon salt
- 1/2 cup chopped walnuts or pecans

Steps:
1. Preheat your oven to 350°F (175°C). Line a muffin tin with paper liners or grease it lightly.
2. In a large mixing bowl, mash the ripe bananas until smooth.
3. Add eggs, honey or maple syrup, applesauce, Greek yogurt, and vanilla extract to the mashed bananas. Mix well until fully combined.
4. Whisk together almond flour, protein powder, baking powder, baking soda, and salt in a separate bowl.
5. Gradually add the dry ingredients to the wet ingredients, stirring until combined. Be careful not to overmix.
6. Fold in the chopped walnuts or pecans gently into the batter.
7. Spoon the batter into the prepared muffin tin, filling each cup about 2/3 full.

8. Bake in the preheated oven for 20-25 minutes, until the tops are golden brown and a toothpick inserted into the center comes clean.
9. Remove the muffins from the oven and let them cool in the tin for a few minutes before transferring them to a wire rack to cool completely.

Nutrition Facts (per muffin):
- Calories: 160
- Total Fat: 9g
    - Saturated Fat: 1g
    - Trans Fat: 0g
- Cholesterol: 31mg
- Sodium: 127mg
- Total Carbohydrate: 15g
    - Dietary Fiber: 2g
    - Sugars: 9g
- Protein: 6g

Egg and Veggie Breakfast Tacos
Cooking Time: 15 minutes
Serving: 4 tacos
Materials:
- Four large eggs
- One tablespoon olive oil
- 1/2 cup diced bell peppers (any color)
- 1/2 cup diced onions
- 1/2 cup diced tomatoes
- 1/2 cup diced mushrooms
- Salt and pepper to taste
- Four small flour tortillas
- 1/4 cup shredded cheddar cheese (optional)
- Salsa, avocado slices, and cilantro for garnish (optional)

Steps:
1. **Prepare the Vegetables:** Heat olive oil in a skillet over medium heat. Add diced bell peppers, onions, tomatoes, and mushrooms. Sauté until vegetables are tender, about 5-7 minutes. Season with salt and pepper to taste.
2. **Scramble the Eggs:** Crack the eggs and whisk them together in a separate bowl. Push the sautéed vegetables to one side of the skillet and pour the beaten eggs into the other. Cook, stirring occasionally, until the eggs are scrambled and cooked through, about 2-3 minutes.

3. **Warm the Tortillas:** While cooking eggs, heat the flour tortillas in a separate skillet or microwave until warm and pliable.
4. **Assemble the Tacos:** Divide the scrambled eggs and sautéed vegetables evenly among the warm tortillas. If using, sprinkle shredded cheddar cheese on top of the eggs. Garnish with salsa, avocado slices, and cilantro if desired.
5. **Serve:** Serve immediately and enjoy your delicious Egg and Veggie Breakfast Tacos!

Nutrition Facts (per serving):
- Calories: 220
- Total Fat: 11g
- Saturated Fat: 3g
- Cholesterol: 195mg
- Sodium: 380mg
- Total Carbohydrates: 20g
- Dietary Fiber: 2g
- Sugars: 3g
- Protein: 11g

Broccoli and Cheese Egg Muffins
Cooking Time: 25 minutes
 Serving: 6 muffins
Materials:
- Six large eggs
- 1 cup chopped broccoli florets
- 1/2 cup shredded cheddar cheese
- 1/4 cup diced bell peppers (any color)
- 1/4 cup diced onions
- Salt and pepper to taste
- Cooking spray or muffin liners

Steps:
1. Preheat your oven to 375°F (190°C). Grease a muffin tin with cooking spray or line it with muffin liners.
2. In a bowl, beat the eggs until well combined. Season with salt and pepper to taste.
3. Stir in the chopped broccoli, shredded cheddar cheese, bell peppers, and onions into the egg mixture. Make sure all ingredients are evenly distributed.

4. Pour the egg mixture evenly into the muffin cups, filling each cup about 3/4 full.
5. Place the muffin tin in the preheated oven and bake for about 20-25 minutes, or until the egg muffins are set and slightly golden on top.
6. Once done, remove the muffin tin from the oven and let the egg muffins cool for a few minutes before serving.
7. Serve warm and enjoy!

Nutrition Facts:

- Serving Size: 1 muffin
- Calories: 120
- Total Fat: 8g
- Saturated Fat: 3g
- Cholesterol: 192mg
- Sodium: 140mg
- Total Carbohydrates: 3g
- Dietary Fiber: 1g
- Sugars: 1g
- Protein: 9g

Chicken Caesar Salad Wrap

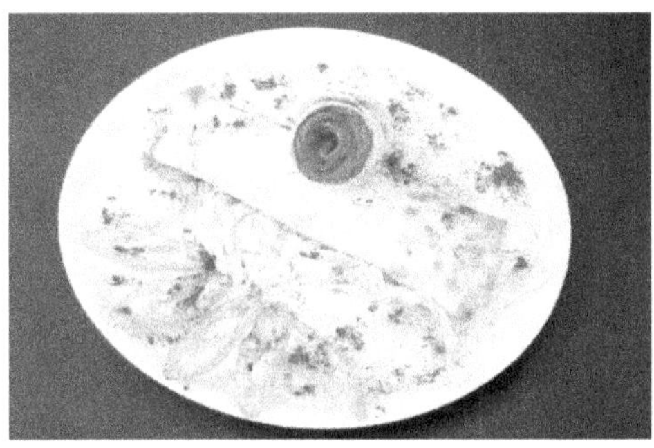

Cooking Time: 20 minutes
 Serving: 4 wraps
Materials:
- Two boneless, skinless chicken breasts
- Salt and pepper to taste
- Four large flour tortillas
- 2 cups romaine lettuce, chopped
- 1/2 cup grated Parmesan cheese
- 1/2 cup Caesar dressing
- 1/4 cup croutons, crushed
- Optional: additional toppings such as cherry tomatoes or bacon bits

Steps:
1. Season the chicken breasts with salt and pepper on both sides.
2. Heat a skillet over medium heat and lightly grease it with oil.
3. Cook the chicken breasts in the skillet for 6-7 minutes per side until cooked and no longer pink in the center. Remove from heat and let them rest for a few minutes before slicing.
4. Lay out the flour tortillas on a clean surface.
5. Divide the chopped romaine lettuce evenly among the tortillas, placing it in the center.

6. Slice the cooked chicken breasts into thin strips and distribute them evenly among the tortillas on top of the lettuce.
7. Sprinkle-grated Parmesan cheese over the chicken.
8. Drizzle Caesar dressing over the chicken and lettuce.
9. Sprinkle crushed croutons over the top.
10. Add toppings, such as cherry tomatoes or bacon bits if desired.
11. Carefully fold the sides of each tortilla inward, then roll tightly to form a wrap.
12. Serve immediately or wrap tightly in foil or parchment paper for later enjoyment.

Nutrition Facts (per serving):
- Calories: 350
- Total Fat: 18g
  - Saturated Fat: 5g
  - Trans Fat: 0g
- Cholesterol: 65mg
- Sodium: 800mg
- Total Carbohydrates: 21g
  - Dietary Fiber: 2g
  - Sugars: 2g
- Protein: 25g

Quinoa Salad with Roasted Vegetables
Cooking Time: 30 minutes
Serving: 4
Materials:
- 1 cup quinoa, rinsed
- 2 cups water or vegetable broth
- One medium red bell pepper, diced
- One medium yellow bell pepper, diced
- One medium zucchini, sliced
- One medium red onion, thinly sliced
- Two tablespoons of olive oil
- Salt and pepper to taste
- 1/4 cup chopped fresh parsley

Steps:
1. Preheat your oven to 400°F (200°C).
2. Bring the water or vegetable broth to a boil in a medium saucepan. Add the rinsed quinoa, reduce the heat to low, cover, and let simmer for about

15 minutes, or until the quinoa is cooked and the liquid is absorbed. Remove from heat and let it sit covered for 5 minutes, then fluff with a fork.

3. While the quinoa is cooking, spread the diced bell peppers, sliced zucchini, and thinly sliced red onion on a baking sheet. Drizzle with olive oil and season with salt and pepper. Toss to coat evenly.
4. Roast the vegetables in the oven for about 15-20 minutes, or until they are tender and slightly caramelized, stirring halfway through.
5. In a large mixing bowl, combine the cooked quinoa and roasted vegetables. Toss gently to mix.
6. Sprinkle the chopped fresh parsley over the salad and toss again.
7. Serve the quinoa salad warm or at room temperature.

Nutrition Facts (per serving):
- Calories: 250
- Total Fat: 8g
    - Saturated Fat: 1g
- Cholesterol: 0mg
- Sodium: 20mg
- Total Carbohydrates: 38g
    - Dietary Fiber: 6g
    - Sugars: 5g
- Protein: 7g

Turkey and Avocado Lettuce Wraps

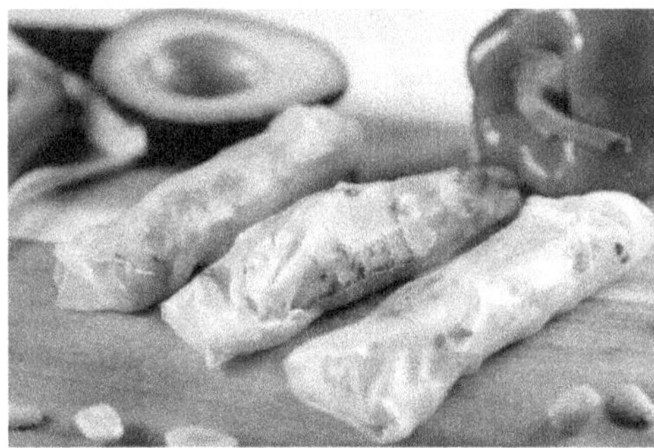

Cooking Time: 15 minutes
 Servings: 4
Materials:
- 1 lb ground turkey

- Two avocados, diced
- One small red onion, finely chopped
- One bell pepper, diced
- Two cloves garlic, minced
- One tablespoon of olive oil
- Salt and pepper to taste
- Eight large lettuce leaves (such as iceberg or butter lettuce)
- Optional toppings: diced tomatoes, shredded cheese, hot sauce

Steps:

1. Heat olive oil in a large skillet over medium heat.
2. Add minced garlic and chopped red onion to the skillet. Sauté until fragrant and translucent, about 2 minutes.
3. Add ground turkey to the skillet. Break it apart with a spatula until browned and cooked about 5-7 minutes.
4. Once the turkey is cooked, add diced bell pepper to the skillet. Cook for 2-3 minutes until the bell pepper is slightly softened.
5. Season the turkey mixture with salt and pepper to taste.
6. Remove the skillet from heat and let the mixture cool slightly.
7. Wash and dry the lettuce leaves, then lay them on a clean surface.
8. Spoon the turkey mixture onto each lettuce leaf, dividing it evenly among them.
9. Top each lettuce wrap with diced avocado.
10. Add toppings such as diced tomatoes, shredded cheese, or hot sauce if desired.
11. Roll up the lettuce leaves, tucking in the sides as you form wraps.
12. Serve immediately and enjoy!

Nutrition Facts (per serving):

- Calories: 320
- Total Fat: 18g
    - Saturated Fat: 4g
    - Trans Fat: 0g
- Cholesterol: 80mg
- Sodium: 250mg
- Total Carbohydrate: 10g
    - Dietary Fiber: 6g
    - Sugars: 2g
- Protein: 28g

Greek Chicken Bowls with Tzatziki Sauce
Cooking Time: 30 minutes
 Servings: 4
Materials:

- 1 lb chicken breasts, cut into bite-sized pieces
- Two tablespoons of olive oil
- One teaspoon dried oregano
- One teaspoon of dried thyme
- Salt and pepper to taste
- 2 cups cooked quinoa
- One cucumber, diced
- 1 cup cherry tomatoes, halved
- 1/2 red onion, thinly sliced
- 1/4 cup crumbled feta cheese
- 1/4 cup chopped fresh parsley
- Four whole wheat pitas warmed

For the Tzatziki Sauce:

- 1 cup Greek yogurt
- 1/2 cucumber, grated and squeezed to remove excess moisture
- Two cloves garlic, minced
- One tablespoon of lemon juice
- One tablespoon chopped fresh dill
- Salt and pepper to taste

Steps:

1. **Marinate the Chicken:** In a bowl, combine the chicken pieces with olive oil, dried oregano, thyme, salt, and pepper. Toss until the chicken is evenly coated. Let it marinate for at least 15 minutes.
2. **Prepare the Tzatziki Sauce:** In another bowl, mix Greek yogurt, grated cucumber, minced garlic, lemon juice, chopped fresh dill, salt, and pepper. Stir until well combined. Refrigerate until ready to use.
3. **Cook the Chicken:** Heat a skillet over medium-high heat. Add the marinated chicken pieces and cook until golden brown and cooked through about 6-8 minutes.
4. **Assemble the Bowls:** Divide cooked quinoa among four bowls. Top each bowl with cooked chicken, diced cucumber, cherry tomatoes, sliced red onion, crumbled feta cheese, and chopped fresh parsley.
5. **Serve:** Serve the Greek chicken bowls with warm whole wheat pitas and a generous dollop of tzatziki sauce on top.

Nutrition Facts (per serving):

- Calories: 480
- Total Fat: 15g
- Saturated Fat: 4g
- Cholesterol: 90mg
- Sodium: 450mg
- Total Carbohydrates: 44g
- Dietary Fiber: 6g
- Sugars: 6g
- Protein: 42g

Taco Salad with Ground Turkey and Black Beans

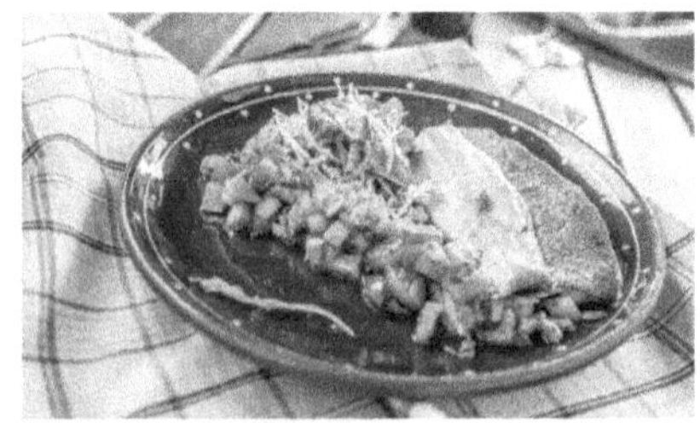

Cooking Time: 25 minutes
 Servings: 4
Materials:
- 1 pound ground turkey
- One can (15 ounces) black beans, rinsed and drained
- One tablespoon of olive oil
- One packet of taco seasoning
- 4 cups mixed salad greens
- 1 cup cherry tomatoes, halved
- One avocado, diced
- 1/2 cup shredded cheddar cheese
- 1/4 cup chopped cilantro
- 1/4 cup sliced black olives
- 1/4 cup diced red onion
- One lime, cut into wedges
- Tortilla chips (optional for serving)

Steps:

1. **Cook Ground Turkey:** Heat olive oil over medium heat in a large skillet. Add ground turkey and cook until browned, breaking it apart with a spoon as it cooks. Drain any excess fat.
2. **Season Turkey:** Sprinkle taco seasoning over the cooked turkey, stirring well to combine. Add black beans to the skillet and stir until heated, about 3-4 minutes. Remove from heat and set aside.
3. **Prepare Salad Base:** In a large mixing bowl, combine mixed salad greens, cherry tomatoes, avocado, shredded cheddar cheese, chopped cilantro, sliced black olives, and diced red onion. Toss gently to combine.
4. **Assemble Salad:** Divide the salad mixture among serving plates or bowls. Top each portion with a generous spoonful of the seasoned ground turkey and black bean mixture.
5. **Garnish and Serve:** Garnish each salad with a lime wedge for squeezing over the top. Serve immediately, with tortilla chips on the side if desired.

Nutrition Facts (per serving):
- **Calories:** 425 kcal
- **Total Fat:** 20g
    - Saturated Fat: 5g
    - Trans Fat: 0g
- **Cholesterol:** 80mg
- **Sodium:** 670mg
- **Total Carbohydrates:** 31g
    - Dietary Fiber: 11g
    - Sugars: 4g
- **Protein:** 32g

Spinach and Feta Stuffed Chicken Breast

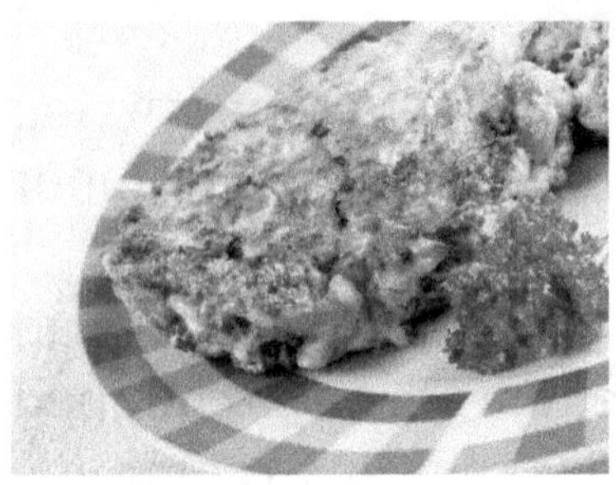

Cooking Time: 40 minutes
 Serving: 4
Materials:
- Four boneless, skinless chicken breasts
- 2 cups fresh spinach, chopped
- 1/2 cup feta cheese, crumbled
- Two cloves garlic, minced
- One tablespoon of olive oil
- Salt and pepper to taste
- Toothpicks or kitchen twine

Steps:
1. Preheat your oven to 375°F (190°C).
2. In a skillet, heat olive oil over medium heat. Add minced garlic and cook for about 1 minute until fragrant.
3. Add chopped spinach to the skillet and cook until wilted, about 3-4 minutes. Season with salt and pepper to taste. Remove from heat and let it cool slightly.
4. Butterfly each chicken breast by slicing horizontally through the center, but not cutting all the way through, to create a pocket.
5. Stuff each chicken breast with equal amounts of the cooked spinach and crumbled feta cheese.
6. Use toothpicks or kitchen twine to secure the opening of each chicken breast to keep the filling inside.
7. Season the stuffed chicken breasts with salt and pepper.
8. Heat a skillet over medium-high heat and add a little olive oil. Once hot, add the stuffed chicken breasts and sear for 2-3 minutes on each side until golden brown.

9. Transfer the seared chicken breasts to a baking dish and bake in the oven for about 20-25 minutes or until the chicken is cooked and no longer pink in the center.

10.   Once cooked, remove the toothpicks or kitchen twine before serving.

Nutrition Facts (per serving):

- Calories: 280
- Total Fat: 12g
- Saturated Fat: 4g
- Cholesterol: 110mg
- Sodium: 360mg
- Total Carbohydrates: 2g
- Dietary Fiber: 1g
- Sugars: 0g
- Protein: 38g

Bariatric-Friendly Chicken Salad with Grapes and Walnuts

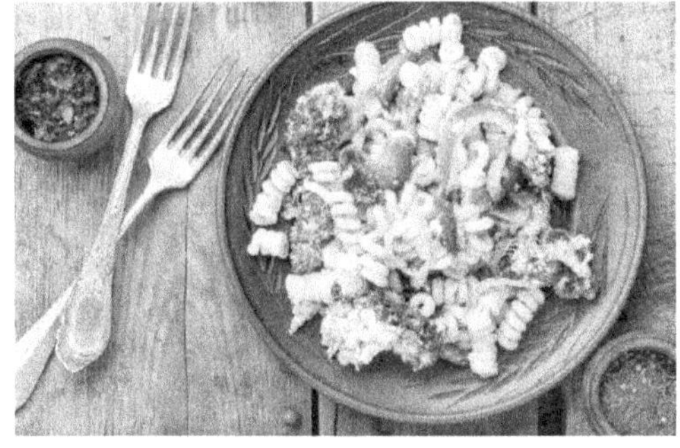

Cooking Time: 20 minutes
Serving: 4
Materials:

- 2 cups cooked chicken breast, diced
- 1 cup seedless grapes, halved
- 1/2 cup walnuts, chopped
- 1/4 cup plain Greek yogurt
- One tablespoon mayonnaise
- One tablespoon of lemon juice
- One tablespoon honey
- Salt and pepper to taste

- Lettuce leaves for serving

Steps:

1. **Prepare Ingredients:** Cook chicken breasts until fully cooked, then dice them into bite-sized pieces. Halve the seedless grapes and chop the walnuts.
2. **Make Dressing:** In a small bowl, mix the Greek yogurt, mayonnaise, lemon juice, and honey until well combined. Season with salt and pepper to taste.
3. **Combine Ingredients:** In a large mixing bowl, combine the diced chicken, halved grapes, and chopped walnuts.
4. **Add Dressing:** Pour the dressing over the chicken, grapes, and walnuts. Gently toss until everything is evenly coated with the dressing.
5. **Serve:** Place lettuce leaves on serving plates or bowls. Spoon the chicken salad mixture onto the lettuce leaves.
6. **Enjoy:** Serve immediately and enjoy your bariatric-friendly chicken salad with grapes and walnuts!

Nutrition Facts (Per Serving):

- Calories: 250
- Total Fat: 12g
- Saturated Fat: 1.5g
- Cholesterol: 60mg
- Sodium: 150mg
- Total Carbohydrates: 11g
- Dietary Fiber: 2g
- Sugars: 8g
- Protein: 25g

Salmon and Quinoa Power Bowl

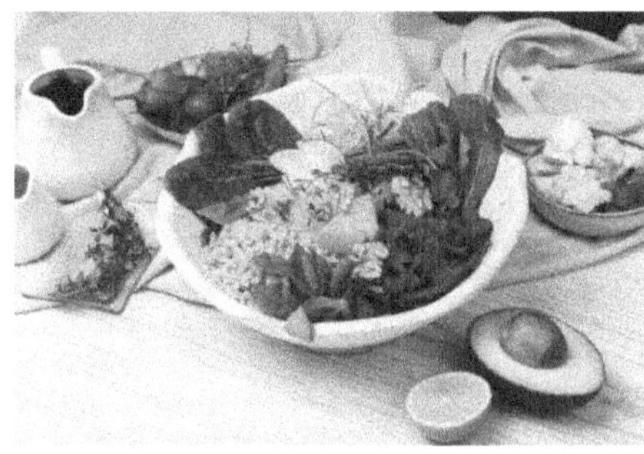

Cooking Time: 30 minutes
 Serving: 2
Materials:
- Two salmon fillets
- 1 cup quinoa
- 2 cups vegetable broth
- 1 cup cherry tomatoes, halved
- One avocado, sliced
- 2 cups baby spinach
- 1/4 cup red onion, thinly sliced
- Two tablespoons of olive oil
- Salt and pepper to taste
- Lemon wedges for serving
- Optional: sesame seeds for garnish

Steps:
1. Rinse the quinoa under cold water. In a medium saucepan, bring the vegetable broth to a boil. Add the rinsed quinoa, reduce heat to low, cover, and simmer for 15-20 minutes or until the quinoa is cooked and the liquid is absorbed. Fluff with a fork and set aside.
2. Preheat the oven to 375°F (190°C). Line a baking sheet with parchment paper or foil.
3. Place the salmon fillets on the prepared baking sheet. Drizzle with olive oil and season with salt and pepper.
4. Bake the salmon in the preheated oven for 12-15 minutes, or until it flakes easily with a fork.
5. While the salmon is baking, assemble the power bowls. Divide the cooked quinoa into two bowls. Top each bowl with baby spinach, cherry tomatoes, avocado slices, and sliced red onion.

6. Once the salmon is cooked, place one fillet in each bowl.
7. Garnish with sesame seeds if desired, and serve with lemon wedges.

Nutrition Facts:
- **Calories:** 480 per serving
- **Protein:** 30g
- **Fat:** 24g
- **Carbohydrates:** 34g
- **Fiber:** 9g
- **Sugar:** 4g
- **Sodium:** 420mg

Veggie-Packed Turkey Chili
Cooking Time: 1 hour
 Serving: 6
Materials:
- One tablespoon of olive oil
- One onion, chopped
- Three cloves garlic, minced
- One red bell pepper, diced
- One green bell pepper, diced
- Two carrots diced
- Two celery stalks, diced
- 1 pound ground turkey
- Two cans (14.5 ounces each) diced tomatoes
- One can (15 ounces) kidney beans, drained and rinsed
- One can (15 ounces) black beans, drained and rinsed
- 2 cups vegetable broth
- Two tablespoons chili powder
- One tablespoon cumin
- One teaspoon paprika
- Salt and pepper to taste
- Optional toppings: shredded cheese, sliced green onions, sour cream, avocado

Steps:
1. Heat olive oil in a large pot over medium heat. Add chopped onion and minced garlic, sauté until fragrant, about 2 minutes.
2. Add diced red and green bell peppers, carrots, and celery to the pot. Cook, stirring occasionally, until vegetables are tender, about 5 minutes.

3. Push the vegetables to one side of the pot and add ground turkey to the empty side. Cook, breaking up the turkey with a spoon, until browned and cooked through, about 5-7 minutes.
4. Stir in diced tomatoes, kidney beans, black beans, vegetable broth, chili powder, cumin, paprika, salt, and pepper. Bring the chili to a simmer.
5. Reduce heat to low and let the chili simmer uncovered for about 30-40 minutes, stirring occasionally, until flavors meld and chili thickens to your desired consistency.
6. Taste and adjust seasoning if needed. Serve hot with your choice of toppings like shredded cheese, sliced green onions, sour cream, or avocado.

Nutrition Facts (per serving):
- Calories: 320
- Total Fat: 10g
- Saturated Fat: 2g
- Cholesterol: 45mg
- Sodium: 760mg
- Total Carbohydrate: 35g
- Dietary Fiber: 11g
- Sugars: 7g
- Protein: 25g

Caprese Salad Skewers with Balsamic Glaze
Cooking Time: 15 minutes
 Serving: 4
Materials:
- 1 pint cherry tomatoes
- 8 ounces fresh mozzarella balls, drained
- Fresh basil leaves
- Balsamic glaze
- Olive oil
- Salt and pepper, to taste
- Wooden skewers

Steps:
1. **Prepare Ingredients:** Rinse cherry tomatoes and pat dry. Drain mozzarella balls. Wash and dry basil leaves.
2. **Assemble Skewers:** Thread one cherry tomato, mozzarella ball, and basil leaf onto each skewer, repeating until all ingredients are used.

3. **Season:** Drizzle assembled skewers with olive oil and sprinkle with salt and pepper to taste.
4. **Serve:** Arrange skewers on a serving platter and drizzle with balsamic glaze before serving.

Nutrition Facts: (per serving)
- **Calories:** 180
- **Total Fat:** 12g
- **Saturated Fat:** 5g
- **Cholesterol:** 25mg
- **Sodium:** 250mg
- **Total Carbohydrates:** 8g
- **Dietary Fiber:** 2g
- **Sugars:** 5g
- **Protein:** 10g

Shrimp and Avocado Salad
Cooking Time: 15 minutes
Servings: 4
Materials:
- 1 pound large shrimp, peeled and deveined
- Two ripe avocados, diced
- 1 cup cherry tomatoes, halved
- 1/4 cup red onion, thinly sliced
- Two tablespoons fresh cilantro, chopped
- 2 tablespoons olive oil
- One tablespoon lime juice
- Salt and pepper to taste
- Optional: mixed greens for serving

Steps:
1. **Cook Shrimp:** Heat olive oil in a large skillet over medium-high heat. Season shrimp with salt and pepper, then add them to the skillet. Cook 2-3 minutes on each side until shrimp turn pink and opaque. Remove from heat and set aside.
2. **Prepare Salad Base:** In a large mixing bowl, combine diced avocados, halved cherry tomatoes, sliced red onion, and chopped cilantro.
3. **Add Shrimp:** Once the shrimp have cooled slightly, add them to the mixing bowl with the other salad ingredients.
4. **Dress Salad:** Drizzle lime juice over the salad mixture and toss gently to combine. Adjust seasoning with additional salt and pepper if needed.

5. **Serve:** Optionally, serve the shrimp and avocado salad over a bed of mixed greens for extra freshness and presentation.

Nutrition Facts (per serving):
- Calories: 280 kcal
- Total Fat: 16g
  - Saturated Fat: 2g
  - Trans Fat: 0g
- Cholesterol: 185mg
- Sodium: 280mg
- Total Carbohydrates: 11g
  - Dietary Fiber: 6g
  - Sugars: 2g
- Protein: 24g

Baked Buffalo Chicken Tenders
Cooking Time: 25 minutes
Serving: 4
Materials:
- 1 pound chicken tenders
- 1 cup breadcrumbs
- 1/2 cup buffalo sauce
- 1/4 cup melted butter
- 1/2 teaspoon garlic powder
- 1/2 teaspoon onion powder
- Salt and pepper to taste
- Cooking spray

Steps:
1. Preheat your oven to 400°F (200°C) and line a baking sheet with parchment paper. Lightly grease the parchment paper with cooking spray.
2. Mix the breadcrumbs, garlic powder, onion powder, salt, and pepper in a shallow bowl.
3. In another bowl, combine the buffalo sauce and melted butter.
4. Dip each chicken tender into the buffalo sauce mixture, then coat it evenly with the breadcrumb mixture. Place the coated tenders on the prepared baking sheet.
5. Once all tenders are coated and placed on the baking sheet, lightly spray the tops with cooking spray. This will help them crisp up in the oven.

6. Bake in the oven for about 20-25 minutes or until the chicken is cooked and the coating is golden brown and crispy.
7. Once done, remove from the oven and let them cool for a few minutes before serving.
8. Serve with your favorite dipping sauce, and enjoy!

Nutrition Facts (per serving):
- Calories: 320
- Total Fat: 14g
- Saturated Fat: 6g
- Cholesterol: 85mg
- Sodium: 980mg
- Total Carbohydrates: 17g
- Dietary Fiber: 1g
- Sugars: 1g
- Protein: 28g

Turkey and Veggie Stir-Fry with Brown Rice
Cooking Time: 25 minutes
 Serving: 4
Materials:
- 1 lb (450g) turkey breast, thinly sliced
- 2 cups mixed vegetables (such as bell peppers, broccoli, carrots, snap peas)
- 2 cups cooked brown rice
- Three tablespoons soy sauce
- Two tablespoons oyster sauce
- One tablespoon sesame oil
- Two cloves garlic, minced
- One teaspoon ginger, grated
- 2 tablespoons vegetable oil
- Salt and pepper to taste
- Optional garnish: sliced green onions, sesame seeds

Steps:
1. **Prepare Ingredients:** Thinly slice the turkey breast and chop the mixed vegetables into bite-sized pieces. Mince the garlic and grate the ginger.
2. **Cook Brown Rice:** If it hasn't been cooked already, prepare the brown rice according to the package instructions. Set aside.
3. **Prepare Sauce:** In a small bowl, mix soy sauce, oyster sauce, sesame oil, minced garlic, and grated ginger. Set aside.

4. **Cook Turkey:** Heat vegetable oil in a large skillet or wok over medium-high heat. Add the sliced turkey breast and cook until browned and cooked, about 5-6 minutes. Remove the turkey from the skillet and set aside.
5. **Stir-Fry Vegetables:** Add a bit more oil to the same skillet if needed. Add the mixed vegetables and stir-fry for 3-4 minutes or until tender yet crisp.
6. **Combine Ingredients:** Return the cooked turkey to the skillet with the vegetables. Pour the prepared sauce over the turkey and vegetables. Stir well to combine and ensure everything is coated in the sauce. Cook for 2-3 minutes, allowing the flavors to meld together.
7. **Serve:** Serve the turkey and veggie stir-fry hot cooked brown rice. If desired, garnish with sliced green onions and sesame seeds.

Nutrition Facts (per serving):
- Calories: 320 kcal
- Protein: 25g
- Carbohydrates: 30g
- Fiber: 4g
- Fat: 10g
- Saturated Fat: 2g
- Cholesterol: 55mg
- Sodium: 800mg
- Potassium: 500mg
- Vitamin A: 50% DV
- Vitamin C: 80% DV
- Calcium: 4% DV
- Iron: 15% DV

Southwest Chicken and Black Bean Quinoa Bowl
Cooking Time: 30 minutes
Serving: 4
Materials:
- 1 cup quinoa, rinsed
- 2 cups chicken broth
- 1 tablespoon olive oil
- 1 pound chicken breast, diced
- One red bell pepper, diced
- One yellow bell pepper, diced
- One can black beans, drained and rinsed
- 1 cup corn kernels

- One teaspoon cumin
- One teaspoon chili powder
- Salt and pepper to taste
- 1 avocado, sliced (for garnish)
- Fresh cilantro, chopped (for garnish)
- Lime wedges (for garnish)

Steps:

1. **Cook Quinoa:** Bring the chicken broth to a boil in a medium saucepan. Add the quinoa, reduce heat to low, cover, and simmer for 15-20 minutes, or until the quinoa is cooked and the liquid is absorbed. Fluff with a fork and set aside.
2. **Prepare Chicken and Vegetables:** Heat olive oil over medium-high heat in a large skillet. Add diced chicken breasts and cook until browned and cooked through, about 5-6 minutes. Remove chicken from skillet and set aside.
3. In the same skillet, add diced bell peppers and cook until slightly softened about 3-4 minutes.
4. **Combine Ingredients:** Return cooked chicken to the skillet. Add black beans, corn kernels, cumin, chili powder, salt, and pepper. Stir well to combine and cook for 2-3 minutes until heated.
5. **Assemble Bowls:** Divide cooked quinoa among serving bowls. Top with the chicken and vegetable mixture.
6. **Garnish:** Garnish each bowl with sliced avocado, chopped cilantro, and lime wedges.

Nutrition Facts (per serving):

- Calories: 420
- Total Fat: 12g
- Saturated Fat: 2g
- Cholesterol: 75mg
- Sodium: 650mg
- Total Carbohydrates: 45g
- Dietary Fiber: 10g
- Sugars: 3g
- Protein: 35g

Cauliflower Crust Pizza with Turkey Pepperoni
Cooking Time: 40 minutes
Serving: 4 servings
Materials:

- One medium-sized cauliflower head, grated
- 1 egg
- 1 cup shredded mozzarella cheese
- One teaspoon dried oregano
- 1/2 teaspoon garlic powder
- 1/4 teaspoon salt
- 1/4 teaspoon black pepper
- 1/2 cup tomato sauce
- 1 cup shredded mozzarella cheese (for topping)
- Turkey pepperoni slices
- Fresh basil leaves (optional, for garnish)

Steps:

1. Preheat your oven to 400°F (200°C).
2. Place the grated cauliflower in a microwave-safe bowl and microwave for 4-5 minutes or until soft. Allow it to cool for a few minutes.
3. Once cooled, transfer the cauliflower to a clean kitchen towel and squeeze out as much moisture as possible.
4. Combine the squeezed cauliflower, egg, 1 cup shredded mozzarella cheese, oregano, garlic powder, salt, and black pepper in a mixing bowl. Mix until well combined.
5. Line a baking sheet with parchment paper and spread the cauliflower mixture onto it, shaping it into a round pizza crust about 1/4 inch thick.
6. Bake the cauliflower crust in the preheated oven for 20-25 minutes or until golden brown and firm to the touch.
7. Remove the crust from the oven and spread the tomato sauce evenly over the crust, leaving a small border around the edges.
8. Sprinkle the remaining shredded mozzarella cheese over the tomato sauce, then arrange the turkey pepperoni slices on top.
9. Return the pizza to the oven and bake for 10-15 minutes until the cheese is melted and bubbly.
10. Once done, remove the pizza from the oven and let it cool for a few minutes before slicing. If desired, garnish with fresh basil leaves.

Nutrition Facts (per serving):

- Calories: 220
- Total Fat: 12g
- Saturated Fat: 6g
- Cholesterol: 70mg
- Sodium: 640mg
- Total Carbohydrates: 9g

- Dietary Fiber: 3g
- Sugars: 3g
- Protein: 19g

Asian Chicken Lettuce Wraps
Cooking Time: 25 minutes
Servings: 4
Materials:
- 1 lb ground chicken
- One tablespoon vegetable oil
- Two cloves garlic, minced
- One tablespoon ginger, minced
- 1/4 cup soy sauce
- Two tablespoons hoisin sauce
- 1 tablespoon rice vinegar
- One tablespoon sesame oil
- One teaspoon Sriracha sauce (optional, adjust to taste)
- 1/4 cup water chestnuts, diced
- Two green onions, thinly sliced
- 1/4 cup chopped peanuts (optional)
- One head iceberg or butter lettuce, leaves separated
- Cooked rice for serving (optional)

Steps:
1. **Prepare Ingredients:** Start by mincing garlic and ginger. Thinly slice the green onions. Dice the water chestnuts and chop the peanuts if you're using them.
2. **Cook Chicken Mixture:** Heat vegetable oil in a large skillet over medium-high heat. Add minced garlic and ginger, and sauté for about 1 minute until fragrant. Add ground chicken to the skillet and cook until browned and cooked through, breaking it up with a spoon as it cooks.
3. **Make Sauce:** In a small bowl, mix soy sauce, hoisin sauce, rice vinegar, sesame oil, and Sriracha sauce. Pour the sauce over the cooked chicken in the skillet.
4. **Add Crunch:** Stir in diced water chestnuts and sliced green onions. Cook for another 2-3 minutes until heated through and well combined.
5. **Serve:** Spoon the chicken mixture into lettuce leaves, garnish with chopped peanuts if desired, and serve immediately. If preferred, serve with cooked rice on the side.

Nutrition Facts (per serving):

- Calories: 275 kcal
- Total Fat: 15g
    - Saturated Fat: 3g
- Cholesterol: 85mg
- Sodium: 822mg
- Total Carbohydrates: 8g
    - Dietary Fiber: 2g
    - Sugars: 3g
- Protein: 27g

Mediterranean Chickpea Salad with Feta

Cooking Time: 15 minutes

Servings: 4

Materials:

- Two cans (15 ounces each) chickpeas, drained and rinsed
- 1 cup cherry tomatoes, halved
- One cucumber, diced
- One red bell pepper, diced
- 1/2 cup red onion, finely chopped
- 1/2 cup Kalamata olives, pitted and halved
- 4 ounces feta cheese, crumbled
- 1/4 cup fresh parsley, chopped
- 1/4 cup extra virgin olive oil
- Two tablespoons lemon juice
- Two cloves garlic, minced
- Salt and pepper to taste

Steps:

1. Combine chickpeas, cherry tomatoes, cucumber, red bell pepper, red onion, olives, feta cheese, and parsley in a large mixing bowl.
2. To make the dressing, whisk together the olive oil, lemon juice, minced garlic, salt, and pepper in a small bowl.
3. Pour the dressing over the chickpea mixture and toss until well combined.
4. Serve immediately or refrigerate for at least 30 minutes to allow the flavors to meld together.

Nutrition Facts (per serving):

- Calories: 320
- Total Fat: 18g
- Saturated Fat: 5g

- Cholesterol: 17mg
- Sodium: 580mg
- Total Carbohydrate: 32g
- Dietary Fiber: 8g
- Sugars: 6g
- Protein: 10g

Bariatric-Friendly Egg Salad Lettuce Wraps
Cooking Time: 15 minutes
 Serving: 4 wraps
Materials:
- Four large lettuce leaves (such as iceberg or romaine)
- Four hard-boiled eggs, chopped
- 1/4 cup Greek yogurt
- One tablespoon Dijon mustard
- 1/4 cup diced celery
- 1/4 cup diced red bell pepper
- Two tablespoons finely chopped red onion
- Salt and pepper to taste
- Optional: 1 tablespoon chopped fresh herbs (such as dill or parsley)

Steps:
1. **Prepare Lettuce Wraps:** Wash and dry the lettuce leaves. Lay them flat on a clean surface.
2. **Make Egg Salad:** In a mixing bowl, combine the chopped hard-boiled eggs, Greek yogurt, Dijon mustard, diced celery, diced red bell pepper, and chopped red onion. Mix well until everything is evenly combined.
3. **Season:** Season the egg salad with salt and pepper to taste. If desired, you can add chopped fresh herbs for extra flavor.
4. **Assemble Wraps:** Spoon the egg salad mixture evenly onto each lettuce leaf.
5. **Wrap:** Carefully fold the sides of the lettuce leaves over the egg salad filling, then roll them up tightly to form wraps.
6. **Serve:** Place the wraps seam-side down on a serving platter. Optionally, you can secure them with toothpicks to hold them together. Serve immediately and enjoy!

Nutrition Facts (per serving):
- Calories: 120
- Total Fat: 7g
- Saturated Fat: 2g

- Cholesterol: 190mg
- Sodium: 220mg
- Total Carbohydrate: 4g
- Dietary Fiber: 1g
- Sugars: 2g
- Protein: 10g

Turkey and Veggie Stuffed Bell Peppers
Cooking Time: 1 hour
 Servings: 4
Materials:
- 4 large bell peppers (any color), halved and seeds removed
- 1 pound ground turkey
- One onion, diced
- Two cloves garlic, minced
- 1 cup cooked quinoa or rice
- 1 cup diced tomatoes
- 1 cup diced zucchini
- 1 cup diced mushrooms
- 1 cup shredded mozzarella cheese
- One tablespoon olive oil
- One teaspoon dried oregano
- One teaspoon dried basil
- Salt and pepper to taste
- Fresh parsley for garnish (optional)

Steps:
1. Preheat your oven to 375°F (190°C).
2. Heat olive oil in a large skillet over medium heat. Add diced onion and minced garlic, and sauté until softened, about 3-4 minutes.
3. Add ground turkey to the skillet, breaking it up with a spoon. Cook until browned, about 5-6 minutes.
4. Stir in diced tomatoes, zucchini, mushrooms, dried oregano, basil, salt, and pepper. Cook for another 5 minutes, allowing the flavors to meld.
5. Remove the skillet from heat and stir in cooked quinoa or rice until well combined.
6. Arrange the halved bell peppers in a baking dish. Spoon the turkey and vegetable mixture evenly into each pepper half.
7. Cover the dish with foil and bake in the oven for 30 minutes.

8. After 30 minutes, remove the foil, sprinkle shredded mozzarella cheese over the stuffed peppers, and return to the oven.
9. Bake for 10-15 minutes or until the cheese is melted and bubbly.
10. Garnish with fresh parsley if desired before serving.

Nutrition Facts:
- **Calories:** Approximately 350 per serving
- **Protein:** 25g
- **Fat:** 15g
- **Carbohydrates:** 25g
- **Fiber:** 5g
- **Sodium:** 450mg

Lentil and Vegetable Soup
Cooking Time: 45 minutes
 Serving: 4
Materials:
- 1 cup dry green lentils, rinsed
- One onion, diced
- Two carrots, diced
- Two stalks celery, diced
- Two cloves garlic, minced
- 1 can (14 oz) diced tomatoes
- 4 cups vegetable broth
- 1 teaspoon cumin
- One teaspoon paprika
- 1/2 teaspoon turmeric
- Salt and pepper to taste
- 2 tablespoons olive oil
- Fresh parsley or cilantro for garnish (optional)

Steps:
1. Heat olive oil in a large pot over medium heat. Add diced onion, carrots, and celery. Sauté for 5-7 minutes until vegetables are softened.
2. Add minced garlic, cumin, paprika, and turmeric to the pot. Stir well and cook for another minute until fragrant.
3. Pour in the vegetable broth and diced tomatoes with their juices. Bring the soup to a boil.
4. Once boiling, add rinsed lentils to the pot. Reduce the heat to low, cover, and let simmer for 25-30 minutes until lentils are tender.

5. Season the soup with salt and pepper to taste. Adjust the seasoning if needed.
6. Serve hot, garnished with fresh parsley or cilantro if desired.

Nutrition Facts:
- **Serving Size:** 1/4 of recipe
- **Calories:** 250
- **Total Fat:** 6g
- **Saturated Fat:** 1g
- **Cholesterol:** 0mg
- **Sodium:** 700mg
- **Total Carbohydrate:** 38g
- **Dietary Fiber:** 14g
- **Total Sugars:** 7g
- **Protein:** 13g

Grilled Chicken Caesar Salad
Cooking Time: 30 minutes
 Serving: 4
Materials:
- Two boneless, skinless chicken breasts
- One head romaine lettuce, washed and chopped
- 1 cup cherry tomatoes, halved
- 1/2 cup croutons
- 1/4 cup grated Parmesan cheese
- Caesar salad dressing
- Salt and pepper to taste
- Olive oil

Steps:
1. Preheat your grill to medium-high heat.
2. Season the chicken breasts with salt, pepper, and olive oil.
3. Grill the chicken breasts for about 6-8 minutes per side or until they reach an internal temperature of 165°F (75°C). Remove from the grill and let them rest for a few minutes before slicing.
4. While the chicken is grilling, prepare the salad. Combine the chopped romaine lettuce, cherry tomatoes, croutons, and grated Parmesan cheese in a large mixing bowl.
5. Once the chicken has rested, slice it thinly.
6. Add the sliced chicken to the salad bowl.

7. Drizzle Caesar salad dressing over the salad, starting with a few tablespoons and adding more to taste.
8. Toss the salad gently to coat everything evenly with the dressing.
9. Serve the Grilled Chicken Caesar Salad immediately, garnished with additional grated Parmesan cheese if desired.

Nutrition Facts (per serving):

- Calories: 280
- Total Fat: 12g
    - Saturated Fat: 3g
    - Trans Fat: 0g
- Cholesterol: 75mg
- Sodium: 480mg
- Total Carbohydrates: 11g
    - Dietary Fiber: 3g
    - Sugars: 3g
- Protein: 30g

Quinoa and Black Bean Stuffed Sweet Potatoes
Cooking Time: 1 hour
Serving: 4
Materials:

- Four medium sweet potatoes
- 1 cup quinoa
- 1 can (15 oz) black beans, drained and rinsed
- One red bell pepper, diced
- One small red onion, diced
- Two cloves garlic, minced
- One teaspoon cumin
- One teaspoon paprika
- Salt and pepper to taste
- Olive oil
- Optional toppings: avocado slices, cilantro, lime wedges, salsa

Steps:

1. Preheat your oven to 400°F (200°C).
2. Wash the sweet potatoes thoroughly and pat them dry. Pierce each sweet potato several times with a fork.
3. Place the sweet potatoes on a baking sheet lined with parchment paper. Drizzle with olive oil and sprinkle with salt. Bake in the preheated oven for 45-60 minutes or until they are tender.

4. While the sweet potatoes are baking, rinse the quinoa under cold water. In a medium saucepan, combine the quinoa with 2 cups of water. Bring to a boil, then reduce the heat to low, cover, and simmer for 15-20 minutes, or until the quinoa is cooked and the water is absorbed. Remove from heat and fluff with a fork.
5. Heat a tablespoon of olive oil over medium heat in a large skillet. Add the diced onion, bell pepper, and sauté until softened, about 5 minutes. Add the minced garlic, cumin, paprika, salt, and pepper, and cook for another minute.
6. Add the cooked quinoa and black beans to the skillet with the vegetables. Stir to combine and cook for 2-3 minutes until heated.
7. Once the sweet potatoes are done baking, remove them from the oven and let them cool slightly. Slice each sweet potato lengthwise down the center, careful not to cut through all the way.
8. Gently fluff the insides of the sweet potatoes with a fork. Spoon the quinoa and black bean mixture into the center of each sweet potato.
9. Serve hot stuffed sweet potatoes garnished with avocado slices, cilantro, lime wedges, or salsa.

Nutrition Facts (per serving):
- Calories: 380
- Total Fat: 5g
- Saturated Fat: 1g
- Cholesterol: 0mg
- Sodium: 320mg
- Total Carbohydrate: 73g
- Dietary Fiber: 12g
- Sugars: 10g
- Protein: 13g

Tuna Salad Stuffed Avocado
Cooking Time: 15 minutes
 Serving: 2
Materials:
- Two ripe avocados
- One can (5 oz) tuna, drained
- Two tablespoons mayonnaise
- One tablespoon Dijon mustard
- One tablespoon lemon juice
- 1/4 cup diced red onion

- 1/4 cup diced celery
- Salt and pepper to taste
- Fresh parsley, chopped (for garnish)

Steps:

1. Cut the avocados in half and remove the pits. Scoop out a little extra flesh from each half to create a larger well for the tuna salad.
2. Combine the drained tuna, mayonnaise, Dijon mustard, lemon juice, diced red onion, and diced celery in a mixing bowl. Mix well until everything is evenly combined.
3. Season the tuna salad with salt and pepper to taste. Adjust the seasoning according to your preference.
4. Spoon the tuna salad mixture into the well of each avocado half, dividing it evenly between them.
5. Garnish the stuffed avocados with freshly chopped parsley.
6. Serve immediately and enjoy!

Nutrition Facts:

- **Serving Size:** 1 stuffed avocado half
- **Calories:** Approximately 230
- **Total Fat:** 18g
    - Saturated Fat: 3g
    - Trans Fat: 0g
- **Cholesterol:** 20mg
- **Sodium:** 260mg
- **Total Carbohydrates:** 7g
    - Dietary Fiber: 4g
    - Sugars: 1g
- **Protein:** 12g

Greek Orzo Salad with Cucumber and Tomato

Cooking Time: 20 minutes

 Serving: 4

Materials:

- 1 cup orzo pasta
- One cucumber, diced
- 1 cup cherry tomatoes, halved
- 1/2 red onion, thinly sliced
- 1/2 cup Kalamata olives, pitted and halved
- 1/4 cup fresh parsley, chopped
- 1/4 cup feta cheese, crumbled

- Three tablespoons extra virgin olive oil
- Two tablespoons lemon juice
- One clove garlic, minced
- Salt and pepper to taste

Steps:
1. Cook the orzo pasta according to package instructions. Drain and rinse with cold water. Set aside to cool.
2. Combine the cooled orzo pasta, diced cucumber, cherry tomatoes, sliced red onion, Kalamata olives, and chopped parsley in a large mixing bowl.
3. Whisk together the extra virgin olive oil, lemon juice, minced garlic, salt, and pepper in a small bowl to make the dressing.
4. Pour the dressing over the orzo salad mixture and toss until evenly coated.
5. Sprinkle crumbled feta cheese on top of the salad.
6. Serve immediately or refrigerate for a few hours to allow the flavors to meld together before serving.

Nutrition Facts (per serving):
- Calories: 280 kcal
- Total Fat: 14g
  - Saturated Fat: 3g
  - Trans Fat: 0g
- Cholesterol: 8mg
- Sodium: 350mg
- Total Carbohydrates: 32g
  - Dietary Fiber: 3g
  - Sugars: 3g
- Protein: 7g

Baked Turkey and Veggie Meatballs served with Marinara Sauce
Cooking Time: 30 minutes
 Servings: 4
Materials:
- 1 pound ground turkey
- 1 cup finely chopped mixed vegetables (such as bell peppers, onions, carrots)
- 1/2 cup breadcrumbs
- 1/4 cup grated Parmesan cheese
- One egg, beaten
- Two cloves garlic, minced

- One teaspoon dried oregano
- One teaspoon dried basil
- Salt and pepper to taste
- 1 1/2 cups marinara sauce
- Fresh parsley, chopped (for garnish)

Steps:

1. Preheat your oven to 400°F (200°C). Line a baking sheet with parchment paper or lightly grease it with oil.
2. Combine the ground turkey, chopped vegetables, breadcrumbs, Parmesan cheese, beaten egg, minced garlic, dried oregano, dried basil, salt, and pepper in a large mixing bowl. Mix well until all ingredients are evenly distributed.
3. Shape the mixture into meatballs, about 1 to 1.5 inches in diameter, and place them on the prepared baking sheet.
4. Bake the meatballs in the oven for 20-25 minutes or until they are cooked and browned outside.
5. While the meatballs are baking, heat the marinara sauce in a saucepan over medium heat until warmed through.
6. Once the meatballs are done, remove them from the oven and let them cool slightly.
7. Serve the baked turkey and veggie meatballs with warm marinara sauce drizzled over the top. Garnish with freshly chopped parsley if desired.

Nutrition Facts:

- **Calories:** 270 kcal
- **Total Fat:** 12g
    - Saturated Fat: 3.5g
    - Trans Fat: 0g
- **Cholesterol:** 110mg
- **Sodium:** 590mg
- **Total Carbohydrates:** 15g
    - Dietary Fiber: 2g
    - Sugars: 4g
- **Protein:** 25g

Baked Lemon Herb Salmon with Asparagus

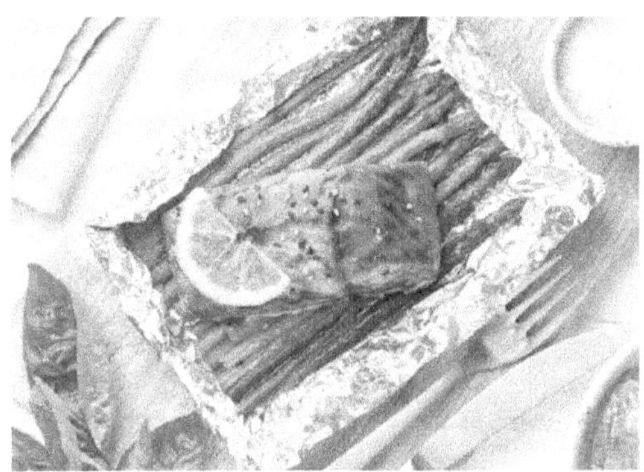

Cooking Time: 25 minutes
 Serving: 4 servings
Materials:

- Four salmon fillets (about 6 ounces each)
- One bunch of asparagus, trimmed
- Two lemons, sliced
- Three tablespoons olive oil
- Two cloves garlic, minced
- One teaspoon of dried thyme
- One teaspoon of dried rosemary
- Salt and black pepper to taste
- Fresh parsley for garnish

Steps:

1. Preheat your oven to 400°F (200°C). Line a baking sheet with parchment paper or aluminum foil for easy cleanup.
2. Place the salmon fillets on one side of the baking sheet, leaving space for the asparagus. Arrange the asparagus next to the salmon.
3. Drizzle the olive oil over the salmon and asparagus. Sprinkle minced garlic, dried thyme, and dried rosemary evenly over the salmon fillets and asparagus.
4. Season with salt and black pepper according to your taste.
5. Place lemon slices over the salmon fillets and asparagus.
6. Bake in the preheated oven for about 15-20 minutes, or until the salmon is cooked, flakes easily with a fork, and the asparagus is tender but still crisp.
7. Once done, remove from the oven and garnish with fresh parsley.

8. Serve hot, with additional lemon slices if desired.

Nutrition Facts:

- **Calories:** Approximately 350 per serving
- **Protein:** Approximately 30g per serving
- **Fat:** Approximately 20g per serving
- **Carbohydrates:** Approximately 10g per serving
- **Fiber:** Approximately 4g per serving

Turkey Taco Stuffed Bell Peppers

Cooking Time: 45 minutes

 Serving: 4 servings

Materials:

- Four large bell peppers (any color), halved and seeds removed
- 1 pound ground turkey
- One tablespoon of olive oil
- One small onion, diced
- Two cloves garlic, minced
- One packet of taco seasoning
- 1 cup cooked rice
- 1 cup black beans, drained and rinsed
- 1 cup corn kernels
- 1 cup salsa
- 1 cup shredded cheddar cheese
- Salt and pepper to taste
- Optional toppings: chopped fresh cilantro, sliced avocado, sour cream

Steps:

1. Preheat your oven to 375°F (190°C). Place the halved bell peppers in a baking dish, cut side up.
2. In a skillet, heat olive oil over medium heat. Add diced onion and minced garlic. Cook until softened, about 2-3 minutes.
3. Add ground turkey to the skillet and cook until browned, breaking it apart with a spatula as it cooks. Drain any excess fat if necessary.
4. Stir in the taco seasoning, cooked rice, black beans, corn, and salsa. Cook for another 5 minutes, allowing the flavors to meld together. Season with salt and pepper to taste.
5. Spoon the turkey taco mixture evenly into each bell pepper half, pressing down gently to pack it in.
6. Cover the baking dish with aluminum foil and bake in the oven for 25-30 minutes or until the peppers are tender.

7. Remove the foil and sprinkle shredded cheddar cheese over the stuffed peppers. Return to the oven and bake uncovered for 5-10 minutes or until the cheese is melted and bubbly.
8. Serve hot, garnished with optional toppings like chopped fresh cilantro, sliced avocado, and sour cream.

Nutrition Facts:
- **Calories:** Approximately 380 per serving
- **Total Fat:** 17g
- **Saturated Fat:** 6g
- **Cholesterol:** 85mg
- **Sodium:** 720mg
- **Total Carbohydrates:** 31g
- **Dietary Fiber:** 6g
- **Total Sugars:** 8g
- **Protein:** 28g

Cauliflower Fried Rice with Shrimp

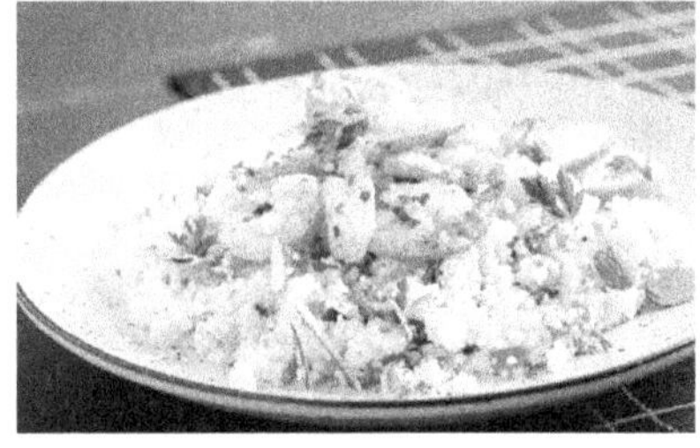

Cooking Time: 20 minutes
Serving: 4 servings
Materials:
- One medium-head cauliflower, grated or finely chopped
- 1 pound shrimp, peeled and deveined
- Two tablespoons of sesame oil
- Two tablespoons soy sauce (or tamari for gluten-free)
- Two cloves garlic, minced
- One small onion, diced
- 1 cup mixed vegetables (carrots, peas, bell peppers), diced
- Two eggs, beaten
- Salt and pepper to taste
- Optional garnish: chopped green onions, sesame seeds

Steps:

1. **Prepare Cauliflower:** Grate the Cauliflower using a box grater or chop it finely in a food processor until it resembles rice grains. Set aside.
2. **Cook the Shrimp:** Heat one tablespoon of sesame oil over medium-high heat in a large skillet or wok. Add the shrimp and cook for 2-3 minutes until pink and cooked. Remove the shrimp from the skillet and set aside.
3. **Sauté Aromatics:** Add the remaining tablespoon of sesame oil to the same skillet. Sauté the garlic and onion until fragrant, about 2 minutes.
4. **Add Vegetables:** Stir in the mixed vegetables and cook for another 3-4 minutes until they are tender-crisp.
5. **Add Cauliflower Rice:** The grated Cauliflower to the skillet, stirring constantly. Cook for about 5 minutes until the Cauliflower is tender but not mushy.
6. **Push Cauliflower to the Side:** Push the cauliflower mixture to one side of the skillet. Pour the beaten eggs onto the empty side of the skillet. Scramble the eggs until cooked through.
7. **Combine Everything:** Once the eggs are cooked, mix them into the cauliflower mixture. Add the cooked shrimp back to the skillet.
8. **Season and Serve:** Drizzle soy sauce over the Cauliflower fried rice and shrimp. Season with salt and pepper to taste. Toss everything together until well combined. Garnish with chopped green onions and sesame seeds if desired.

Nutrition Facts (per serving):
- Calories: 250
- Total Fat: 10g
- Saturated Fat: 2g
- Cholesterol: 220mg
- Sodium: 750mg
- Total Carbohydrates: 14g
- Dietary Fiber: 5g
- Sugars: 6g
- Protein: 26g

Grilled Chicken Breast with Roasted Vegetables
Cooking Time: 40 minutes
Serving: 4 servings
Materials:
- Four boneless, skinless chicken breasts
- Two bell peppers (any color), sliced
- One large red onion, sliced

- Two medium zucchinis, sliced
- 1 cup cherry tomatoes
- Three cloves garlic, minced
- Two tablespoons of olive oil
- One teaspoon dried thyme
- One teaspoon of dried rosemary
- Salt and pepper to taste
- Lemon wedges for serving

Steps:

1. Preheat your grill to medium-high heat.
2. Season the chicken breasts with salt, pepper, half of the minced garlic, thyme, and rosemary.
3. Toss the sliced bell peppers, red onion, zucchini, cherry tomatoes, and the remaining minced garlic with olive oil in a large bowl. Season with salt and pepper to taste.
4. Place the seasoned chicken breasts on the preheated grill. Cook for about 6-8 minutes per side until cooked through and reach an internal temperature of 165°F (75°C).
5. While the chicken is cooking, spread the seasoned vegetables on a baking sheet lined with parchment paper.
6. Place the baking sheet with the vegetables in the oven and roast them for about 20-25 minutes or until tender and slightly caramelized.
7. Remove the chicken from the grill and oven once the chicken is cooked and the vegetables are roasted.
8. Serve the grilled chicken breasts with the roasted vegetables on the side. Squeeze fresh lemon juice over the chicken and vegetables before serving.

Nutrition Facts (per serving):

- Calories: 320 kcal
- Total Fat: 12g
  - Saturated Fat: 2g
  - Trans Fat: 0g
- Cholesterol: 90mg
- Sodium: 280mg
- Total Carbohydrates: 12g
  - Dietary Fiber: 3g
  - Sugars: 6g
- Protein: 40g
- Vitamin D: 5%

- Calcium: 6%
- Iron: 15%
- Potassium: 20%

Bariatric-Friendly Zucchini Lasagna

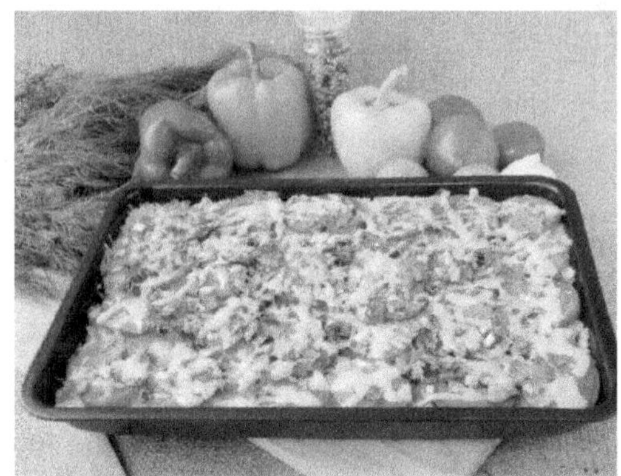

Cooking Time: 1 hour 15 minutes
Serving: 4
Materials:
- Three medium zucchinis, sliced thinly lengthwise
- 1 cup low-fat ricotta cheese
- 1 cup marinara sauce
- 1 cup shredded mozzarella cheese
- 1/4 cup grated Parmesan cheese
- One tablespoon of olive oil
- Two cloves garlic, minced
- One teaspoon dried oregano
- One teaspoon dried basil
- Salt and pepper to taste

Steps:
1. Preheat your oven to 375°F (190°C).
2. In a skillet, heat olive oil over medium heat. Add minced garlic and sauté until fragrant, about 1-2 minutes.
3. Add marinara sauce to the skillet along with dried oregano, dried basil, salt, and pepper. Stir well and let it simmer for 5-7 minutes.
4. Mix ricotta cheese with half of the shredded mozzarella cheese and half of the grated Parmesan cheese in a separate bowl. Set aside.
5. Take a baking dish and spread a thin layer of the marinara sauce mixture on the bottom.

6. Arrange a layer of sliced zucchini over the sauce.
7. Spread half of the ricotta cheese mixture over the zucchini layer.
8. Repeat the layers: marinara sauce, zucchini slices, and the remaining ricotta cheese mixture.
9. Finish with a final layer of marinara sauce on top.
10. Sprinkle the remaining shredded mozzarella and Parmesan cheese on top.
11. Cover the baking dish with foil and cook in the oven for 40 minutes.
12. Remove the foil and bake for 10-15 minutes until the cheese is bubbly and golden brown.
13. Let the lasagna cool for a few minutes before serving.

Nutrition Facts (per serving):

- Calories: 235
- Total Fat: 12g
  - Saturated Fat: 5g
- Cholesterol: 35mg
- Sodium: 580mg
- Total Carbohydrates: 13g
  - Dietary Fiber: 3g
  - Sugars: 6g
- Protein: 18g

Quinoa and Black Bean Enchilada Bake
Cooking Time: 45 minutes
 Servings: 6
Materials:

- 1 cup quinoa, rinsed and drained
- One can (15 oz) black beans, rinsed and drained
- One can (15 oz) enchilada sauce
- 1 cup corn kernels (fresh, frozen, or canned)
- One bell pepper, diced
- One onion, diced
- Two cloves garlic, minced
- One teaspoon ground cumin
- One teaspoon chili powder
- Salt and pepper to taste
- 1 cup shredded cheese (Mexican blend or cheddar)
- Optional toppings: chopped cilantro, diced avocado, sour cream

Steps:

1. Preheat your oven to 375°F (190°C). Grease a 9x13-inch baking dish.
2. In a medium saucepan, combine quinoa and 2 cups of water. Bring to a boil, then reduce heat to low. Cover and simmer for about 15 minutes, until quinoa is cooked and water is absorbed.
3. In a large skillet, heat oil over medium heat. Add diced onion and bell pepper, and sauté until softened about 5 minutes. Add minced garlic, ground cumin, and chili powder, and cook for another minute until fragrant.
4. Stir in cooked quinoa, black beans, corn, and enchilada sauce. Season with salt and pepper to taste. Cook for a few more minutes until heated through.
5. Transfer the quinoa and black bean mixture to the prepared baking dish. Spread it out evenly.
6. Sprinkle shredded cheese over the top of the mixture.
7. Cover the baking dish with foil and bake in the oven for 20-25 minutes or until the cheese is melted and bubbly.
8. Remove from the oven and let it cool for a few minutes before serving.
9. Serve hot, topped with optional toppings like chopped cilantro, diced avocado, and sour cream.

Nutrition Facts (per serving):
- Calories: 320
- Total Fat: 9g
- Saturated Fat: 4g
- Cholesterol: 20mg
- Sodium: 850mg
- Total Carbohydrates: 47g
- Dietary Fiber: 9g
- Sugars: 6g
- Protein: 15g

Turkey and Veggie Meatloaf with Mashed Cauliflower
Cooking Time: 1 hour
 Serving: 4
Materials:
- 1 pound ground turkey
- 1 cup grated zucchini
- 1 cup grated carrot
- 1/2 cup diced onion
- Two cloves garlic, minced

- 1/4 cup breadcrumbs
- 1/4 cup grated Parmesan cheese
- One egg
- One tablespoon Worcestershire sauce
- One teaspoon dried thyme
- Salt and pepper to taste
- Cooking spray

For Mashed Cauliflower:
- One large head cauliflower, cut into florets
- Two cloves garlic, minced
- Two tablespoons butter
- 1/4 cup milk or cream
- Salt and pepper to taste
- Chopped parsley for garnish (optional)

Steps:
1. Preheat your oven to 375°F (190°C). Grease a loaf pan with cooking spray and set aside.
2. In a large mixing bowl, combine the ground turkey, grated zucchini, grated carrot, diced onion, minced garlic, breadcrumbs, Parmesan cheese, egg, Worcestershire sauce, dried thyme, salt, and pepper. Mix until well combined.
3. Transfer the turkey mixture to the prepared loaf pan, pressing it down evenly.
4. Bake in the oven for 45-50 minutes until the meatloaf is cooked and the top is golden brown.
5. While the meatloaf is baking, prepare the mashed Cauliflower. Steam or boil the cauliflower florets and minced garlic until they are tender, about 10-15 minutes.
6. Drain the Cauliflower and garlic, then transfer them to a large mixing bowl. Add the butter and milk or cream. Use a potato masher or immersion blender to mash the Cauliflower until smooth and creamy. Season with salt and pepper to taste.
7. Once the meatloaf is cooked, remove it from the oven and let it rest for a few minutes before slicing.
8. Serve turkey and veggie meatloaf slices with a generous scoop of mashed Cauliflower. If desired, garnish with chopped parsley.

Nutrition Facts (per serving):
- Calories: 320
- Total Fat: 15g

- Saturated Fat: 7g
- Cholesterol: 140mg
- Sodium: 400mg
- Total Carbohydrates: 15g
- Dietary Fiber: 4g
- Sugars: 5g
- Protein: 30g

Lemon Garlic Shrimp Skewers with Quinoa

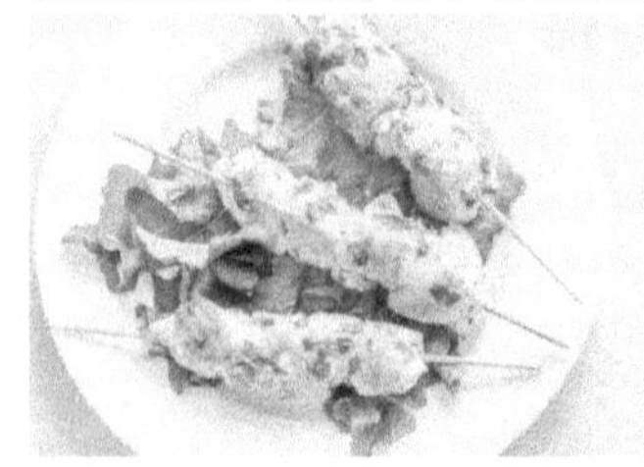

Cooking Time: 25 minutes
Servings: 4
Materials:
- 1 pound large shrimp, peeled and deveined
- Three cloves garlic, minced
- Two tablespoons olive oil
- Zest and juice of 1 lemon
- One teaspoon dried oregano
- Salt and pepper to taste
- 2 cups cooked quinoa
- Wooden skewers, soaked in water for 30 minutes

Steps:
1. Combine minced garlic, olive oil, lemon zest, lemon juice, dried oregano, salt, and pepper in a bowl.
2. Add the peeled and deveined shrimp to the marinade and toss to coat evenly. Let it marinate for about 15 minutes.
3. Preheat your grill or grill pan over medium-high heat.
4. Thread the marinated shrimp onto the soaked wooden skewers.
5. Grill the shrimp skewers for 2-3 minutes per side until they are cooked and have a nice char.
6. While the shrimp are grilling, reheat the cooked quinoa.
7. Serve the grilled shrimp skewers over a bed of warm quinoa.
8. Garnish with fresh lemon slices and chopped parsley if desired.

9. Enjoy your **Lemon Garlic Shrimp Skewers with Quinoa**!
Nutrition Facts:
Note: Nutritional values may vary depending on the ingredients used.
- Serving Size: 1/4 of recipe
- Calories: Approximately 280
- Total Fat: 9g
- Saturated Fat: 1.5g
- Cholesterol: 215mg
- Sodium: 420mg
- Total Carbohydrates: 19g
- Dietary Fiber: 2g
- Sugars: 0g
- Protein: 27g

Beef and Broccoli Stir-Fry with Brown Rice
Cooking Time: 30 minutes
 Servings: 4
Materials:
- 1 pound flank steak, thinly sliced
- 2 cups broccoli florets
- One tablespoon vegetable oil
- Three cloves garlic, minced
- One teaspoon ginger, minced
- 1/4 cup soy sauce
- Two tablespoons oyster sauce
- One tablespoon brown sugar
- One tablespoon cornstarch dissolved in 2 tablespoons water
- Cooked brown rice for serving
- Sesame seeds and sliced green onions for garnish

Steps:
1. **Marinate the beef:** In a bowl, combine thinly sliced flank steak with minced garlic, ginger, soy sauce, and oyster sauce. Let it marinate for at least 15 minutes.
2. **Cook the brown rice:** Prepare brown rice according to package instructions. Keep it warm.
3. **Prepare the broccoli:** Blanch the broccoli florets in boiling water for about 2 minutes, then drain and set aside.

4. **Stir-fry the beef:** Heat vegetable oil in a large skillet or wok over medium-high heat. Add the marinated beef and stir-fry for 3-4 minutes until cooked. Remove the beef from the skillet and set aside.
5. **Cook the sauce:** In the same skillet, add a bit more oil if needed. Stir in minced garlic and cook for 30 seconds. Add soy sauce, oyster sauce, and brown sugar. Stir well to combine.
6. **Thicken the sauce:** Pour the dissolved cornstarch into the skillet, stirring constantly until the sauce thickens.
7. **Combine everything:** Add the cooked beef and blanched broccoli back into the skillet. Toss everything together until well coated in the sauce.
8. **Serve:** Serve the beef and broccoli stir-fry hot over brown rice. If desired, garnish with sesame seeds and sliced green onions.

Nutrition Facts (per serving):
- Calories: 350
- Total Fat: 12g
- Saturated Fat: 4g
- Cholesterol: 75mg
- Sodium: 850mg
- Total Carbohydrates: 25g
- Dietary Fiber: 3g
- Sugars: 6g
- Protein: 30g

Baked Parmesan Crusted Chicken Tenders
Cooking Time: 25 minutes
Servings: 4
Materials:
- 1 pound chicken tenders
- 1 cup grated Parmesan cheese
- 1/2 cup breadcrumbs
- One teaspoon garlic powder
- One teaspoon paprika
- 1/2 teaspoon salt
- 1/4 teaspoon black pepper
- Two eggs, beaten
- Cooking spray

Steps:
1. Preheat your oven to 400°F (200°C). Line a baking sheet with parchment paper and lightly coat it with cooking spray.

2. In a shallow bowl, mix the grated Parmesan cheese, breadcrumbs, garlic powder, paprika, salt, and black pepper.
3. Dip each chicken tender into the beaten eggs, then dredge it in the Parmesan breadcrumb mixture, pressing gently to adhere the coating to the chicken.
4. Place the coated chicken tenders onto the prepared baking sheet, leaving a little space between each piece.
5. Lightly spray the tops of the chicken tenders with cooking spray. This will help them turn golden brown and crispy in the oven.
6. Bake in the oven for about 20-25 minutes or until the chicken is cooked and the coating is crispy and golden brown.
7. Serve hot with your favorite dipping sauce or alongside a fresh salad.

Nutrition Facts (per serving):

- Calories: 320
- Total Fat: 15g
  - Saturated Fat: 6g
  - Trans Fat: 0g
- Cholesterol: 170mg
- Sodium: 800mg
- Total Carbohydrates: 9g
  - Dietary Fiber: 1g
  - Sugars: 1g
- Protein: 35g

Stuffed Portobello Mushrooms with Spinach and Cheese
Cooking Time: 30 minutes
 Servings: 4
Materials:

- Four large Portobello mushrooms
- 2 cups fresh spinach, chopped
- 1 cup ricotta cheese
- 1/2 cup grated Parmesan cheese
- Two cloves garlic, minced
- One tablespoon olive oil
- Salt and pepper to taste
- 1/4 teaspoon red pepper flakes (optional)
- Fresh parsley for garnish

Steps:

1. Preheat your oven to 375°F (190°C). Clean the Portobello mushrooms with a damp cloth or paper towel. Remove the stems and gently scrape out the gills with a spoon. Place the mushrooms on a baking sheet lined with parchment paper.
2. In a skillet, heat the olive oil over medium heat. Add minced garlic and sauté for 1-2 minutes until fragrant.
3. Add chopped spinach to the skillet and cook until wilted, about 3-4 minutes. Season with salt, pepper, and red pepper flakes if using. Remove from heat and let it cool slightly.
4. Mix the cooked spinach with ricotta cheese and grated Parmesan in a mixing bowl until evenly combined.
5. Stuff each Portobello mushroom with the spinach and cheese mixture, dividing it evenly among the mushrooms.
6. Bake in the oven for 20-25 minutes or until the mushrooms are tender and the filling is lightly golden.
7. Once done, remove it from the oven and let it cool for a few minutes. Garnish with fresh parsley before serving.

Nutrition Facts:
- *Serving Size:* 1 stuffed mushroom
- *Calories:* 150
- *Total Fat:* 8g
- *Saturated Fat:* 4g
- *Cholesterol:* 20mg
- *Sodium:* 250mg
- *Total Carbohydrates:* 9g
- *Dietary Fiber:* 2g
- *Sugars:* 3g
- *Protein:* 12g

Turkey and Spinach Spaghetti Squash Boats
Cooking Time: 1-hour **Servings:** 4
Materials:
- Two medium spaghetti squash
- 1 pound ground turkey
- One small onion, diced
- Two cloves garlic, minced
- 1 cup spinach, chopped
- 1 cup marinara sauce
- One teaspoon Italian seasoning

- Salt and pepper to taste
- Olive oil
- Grated Parmesan cheese (optional for serving)

Steps:

1. Preheat your oven to 400°F (200°C).
2. Cut the spaghetti squash in half lengthwise and scoop out the seeds. Drizzle the cut sides with olive oil and season with salt and pepper.
3. Place the squash halves cut side down on a baking sheet lined with parchment paper. Bake for 40-45 minutes until the squash is tender and easily pierced with a fork.
4. While the squash is baking, heat a bit of olive oil in a large skillet over medium heat. Add the diced onion, minced garlic, and sauté until softened and fragrant, about 2-3 minutes.
5. Add the ground turkey to the skillet, breaking it apart with a spoon, and cook until browned and cooked through about 5-7 minutes.
6. Stir in the chopped spinach and cook until wilted about 2 minutes.
7. Add the marinara sauce and Italian seasoning to the skillet, stirring to combine. Let the mixture simmer for another 5 minutes to allow the flavors to meld together. Season with salt and pepper to taste.
8. Once the spaghetti squash is done baking, use a fork to scrape the flesh into strands, leaving about a ½-inch border around the edges to form a "boat."
9. Divide the turkey and spinach mixture among the spaghetti squash boats, filling each evenly.
10. Sprinkle-grated Parmesan cheese on top if desired.
11. Return the stuffed squash boats to the oven and bake for 10-15 minutes, until heated and the cheese is melted and bubbly.
12. Serve hot and enjoy!

Nutrition Facts:

- **Calories:** 320
- **Total Fat:** 12g
- **Saturated Fat:** 3g
- **Cholesterol:** 80mg
- **Sodium:** 580mg
- **Total Carbohydrates:** 24g
- **Dietary Fiber:** 6g
- **Total Sugars:** 10g
- **Protein:** 28g

Bariatric-Friendly Chicken Alfredo with Zucchini Noodles

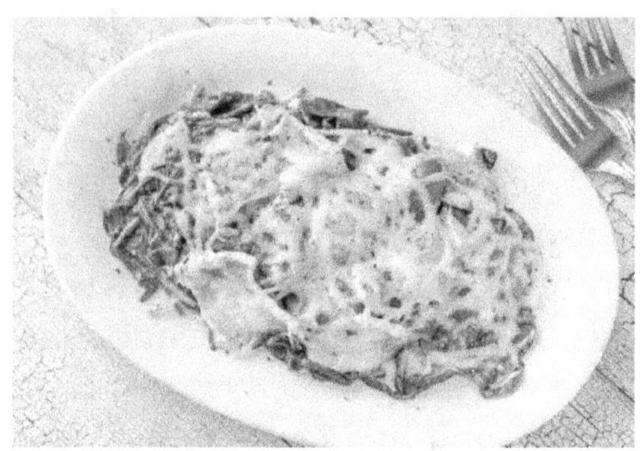

Cooking Time: 25 minutes
 Servings: 2
Materials:
- Two medium-sized zucchinis, spiralized
- Two chicken breasts, thinly sliced
- One tablespoon olive oil
- Two cloves garlic, minced
- 1 cup low-fat milk
- One tablespoon cornstarch
- ¼ cup grated Parmesan cheese
- Salt and pepper to taste
- Fresh parsley for garnish (optional)

Steps:
1. **Prepare Zucchini Noodles:** Spiralize the zucchini using a spiralizer to create noodles. Set aside.
2. **Cook Chicken:** In a skillet, heat olive oil over medium heat. Add minced garlic and cook for about a minute until fragrant. Add thinly sliced chicken breasts to the skillet. Cook until chicken is no longer pink, about 5-6 minutes. Remove chicken from skillet and set aside.
3. **To prepare Alfredo Sauce,** Mix low-fat milk with cornstarch until well combined in the same skillet. Cook over medium heat, stirring constantly, until the mixture thickens, about 3-4 minutes.
4. **Combine Ingredients:** Once the sauce has thickened, add grated Parmesan cheese to the skillet, stirring until the cheese is melted and the sauce is smooth. Season with salt and pepper to taste.

5. **Add Chicken and Zucchini Noodles.** Return the cooked chicken to the skillet with the Alfredo sauce. Stir until the chicken is coated with the sauce. Add the spiralized zucchini noodles to the skillet and toss until the noodles are heated through and coated with the sauce.
6. **Serve:** Divide the chicken alfredo with zucchini noodles evenly between two plates. Garnish with fresh parsley if desired.

Nutrition Facts (per serving):
- Calories: 320
- Total Fat: 12g
- Saturated Fat: 4g
- Cholesterol: 90mg
- Sodium: 410mg
- Total Carbohydrates: 12g
- Dietary Fiber: 2g
- Sugars: 6g
- Protein: 40g

Veggie-packed turkey Meatballs served with Marinara Sauce
Cooking Time: 45 minutes
 Serving: 4 servings
Materials:
- 1 pound ground turkey
- 1 cup grated zucchini
- 1 cup grated carrot
- 1/2 cup breadcrumbs
- 1/4 cup grated Parmesan cheese
- One egg, beaten
- Two cloves garlic, minced
- One teaspoon dried oregano
- One teaspoon dried basil
- Salt and pepper to taste
- 2 cups marinara sauce
- Fresh basil leaves for garnish (optional)

Steps:
1. Preheat your oven to 375°F (190°C). Line a baking sheet with parchment paper or lightly grease it.
2. Combine ground turkey, grated zucchini, grated carrot, breadcrumbs, Parmesan cheese, beaten egg, minced garlic, dried oregano, dried basil,

salt, and pepper in a large mixing bowl. Mix well until all ingredients are evenly incorporated.

3. Place the mixture into golf ball-sized meatballs on the prepared baking sheet.
4. Bake the meatballs in the oven for 20-25 minutes or until they are cooked and lightly browned outside.
5. While the meatballs are baking, heat the marinara sauce in a saucepan over medium heat until warmed through.
6. Once the meatballs are cooked, serve them hot with the marinara sauce spooned over the top. If desired, garnish with fresh basil leaves.

Nutrition Facts:

Note: Nutritional values are approximate and may vary depending on specific ingredients.

- Calories per serving: 320
- Total Fat: 15g
  - Saturated Fat: 4g
  - Trans Fat: 0g
- Cholesterol: 110mg
- Sodium: 820mg
- Total Carbohydrates: 18g
  - Dietary Fiber: 3g
  - Sugars: 7g
- Protein: 28g

Grilled Lemon Herb Chicken Thighs with Cauliflower Mash
Cooking Time: 30 minutes
Serving: 4
Materials:
For Grilled Lemon Herb Chicken Thighs:
- Four boneless, skinless chicken thighs
- Two lemons (juiced and zested)
- Three cloves garlic, minced
- Two tablespoons fresh parsley, chopped
- One tablespoon fresh thyme leaves
- Salt and pepper to taste
- Two tablespoons olive oil

For Cauliflower Mash:
- One large head cauliflower, cut into florets
- Two cloves garlic, minced

- Two tablespoons butter
- 1/4 cup grated Parmesan cheese
- Salt and pepper to taste
- Chopped fresh parsley for garnish (optional)

Steps:

1. **Marinate the Chicken:** In a bowl, combine lemon juice, lemon zest, minced garlic, chopped parsley, thyme leaves, salt, pepper, and olive oil. Place the chicken thighs in the marinade, coating them well. Cover and refrigerate for at least 20 minutes.
2. **Prepare the Cauliflower Mash:** Steam the cauliflower florets and minced garlic until tender, about 10-12 minutes. Drain any excess water. Transfer the cooked Cauliflower and garlic to a food processor. Add butter, Parmesan cheese, salt, and pepper. Blend until smooth and creamy. Adjust seasoning if needed. Keep warm.
3. **Grill the Chicken:** Preheat the grill to medium-high heat. Remove chicken thighs from the marinade, shaking off any excess. Grill the chicken for about 6-8 minutes per side or until fully cooked through and grill marks appear. Make sure the internal temperature reaches 165°F (74°C). Remove from the grill and let rest for a few minutes.
4. **Serve:** Plate the cauliflower mash onto serving plates. Top with grilled lemon herb chicken thighs. Garnish with chopped fresh parsley if desired. Serve hot.

Nutrition Facts (per serving):

Grilled Lemon Herb Chicken Thighs:
- Calories: 250
- Protein: 28g
- Fat: 14g
- Carbohydrates: 3g
- Fiber: 1g

Cauliflower Mash:
- Calories: 120
- Protein: 5g
- Fat: 8g
- Carbohydrates: 10g
- Fiber: 5g

Shrimp and Broccoli Stir-Fry with Quinoa
Cooking Time: 25 minutes
 Serving: 4

Materials:

- 1 cup quinoa
- 1 pound shrimp, peeled and deveined
- 2 cups broccoli florets
- One red bell pepper, sliced
- Three cloves garlic, minced
- One tablespoon ginger, minced
- Two tablespoons soy sauce
- One tablespoon oyster sauce
- One tablespoon sesame oil
- Two tablespoons vegetable oil
- Salt and pepper to taste
- Optional: sliced green onions and sesame seeds for garnish

Steps:

1. **Prepare Quinoa:** Rinse the quinoa under cold water. In a saucepan, combine quinoa and 2 cups of water. Bring to a boil, then reduce heat to low, cover, and simmer for about 15 minutes or until the quinoa is cooked and water is absorbed. Fluff with a fork and set aside.
2. **Prepare Shrimp:** Season the shrimp with salt and pepper. Heat one tablespoon of vegetable oil in a large skillet over medium-high heat. Add the shrimp and cook until pink and opaque, about 2-3 minutes per side. Remove the shrimp from the skillet and set aside.
3. **Stir-Fry Vegetables:** Heat the remaining tablespoon of vegetable oil in the same skillet. Add the garlic and ginger and stir for about 30 seconds until fragrant. Add the broccoli florets and bell pepper slices. Stir-fry for 3-4 minutes until vegetables are tender but still crisp.
4. **Combine Ingredients:** Return the cooked shrimp to the skillet. Add soy sauce, oyster sauce, and sesame oil. Stir to combine all ingredients evenly. Cook for another 2 minutes.
5. **Serve:** Divide the cooked quinoa among serving plates. Top with the shrimp and vegetable stir-fry mixture. Garnish with sliced green onions and sesame seeds if desired.
6. **Enjoy your Shrimp and Broccoli Stir-Fry with Quinoa!**

Nutrition Facts (per serving):

- Calories: 380
- Total Fat: 12g
- Saturated Fat: 2g
- Cholesterol: 175mg
- Sodium: 700mg

- Total Carbohydrates: 38g
- Dietary Fiber: 5g
- Sugars: 3g
- Protein: 30g

Bariatric-Friendly Eggplant Parmesan
Cooking Time: 45 minutes
Servings: 4
Materials:
- One large eggplant, sliced into 1/4-inch rounds
- 1 cup marinara sauce (low-sugar and low-fat, if available)
- 1 cup part-skim mozzarella cheese, shredded
- 1/4 cup grated Parmesan cheese
- 1/4 cup almond flour
- 1/4 cup egg whites
- One teaspoon dried oregano
- One teaspoon dried basil
- Cooking spray
- Salt and pepper to taste

Steps:
1. Preheat the oven to 375°F (190°C). Line a baking sheet with parchment paper and lightly coat it with cooking spray.
2. Combine almond flour, dried oregano, dried basil, and a pinch of salt and pepper in a shallow bowl.
3. In another bowl, beat the egg whites until frothy.
4. Dip each eggplant slice first into the egg whites, allowing excess to drip off, then coat both sides in the almond flour mixture. Place the coated slices on the prepared baking sheet.
5. Bake the eggplant slices in the oven for 20-25 minutes or until golden brown and tender. Remove from the oven and let them cool slightly.
6. In a separate baking dish, spread a thin layer of marinara sauce on the bottom.
7. Arrange half of the baked eggplant slices in a single layer over the marinara sauce.
8. Spoon half of the remaining marinara sauce over the eggplant slices, then sprinkle half of the mozzarella and Parmesan cheese on top.
9. Repeat with another layer of eggplant slices, marinara sauce, and cheese.
10. Bake the assembled eggplant Parmesan in the oven for 15-20 minutes or until the cheese is melted and bubbly.

11.   Let it cool for a few minutes before serving.

Nutrition Facts (per serving):
- Calories: 180
- Total Fat: 8g
  - Saturated Fat: 3.5g
  - Trans Fat: 0g
- Cholesterol: 15mg
- Sodium: 320mg
- Total Carbohydrates: 13g
  - Dietary Fiber: 5g
  - Sugars: 6g
- Protein: 14g

Turkey and Veggie Stuffed Acorn Squash
Cooking Time: 1-hour **Serving:** 4
Materials:
- Two medium acorn squash
- One tablespoon olive oil
- One small onion, diced
- Two cloves garlic, minced
- One bell pepper, diced
- One medium zucchini, diced
- 1 pound ground turkey
- One teaspoon dried thyme
- One teaspoon dried sage
- Salt and pepper to taste
- 1/2 cup shredded mozzarella cheese
- Fresh parsley for garnish (optional)

Steps:
1. Preheat your oven to 400°F (200°C).
2. Slice the acorn squash in half lengthwise and scoop out the seeds. Place the squash halves on a baking sheet and cut side up. Drizzle with olive oil and sprinkle with salt and pepper. Roast in the oven for 30-40 minutes or until the squash is tender when pierced with a fork.
3. While the squash is roasting, heat olive oil in a large skillet over medium heat. Add the diced onion and garlic, and sauté until softened, about 2-3 minutes.
4. Add the diced bell pepper and zucchini to the skillet and cook for 3-4 minutes until they soften.

5. Push the vegetables to the side of the skillet and add the ground turkey to the center. Cook, breaking it apart with a spoon, until the turkey is browned and cooked through.
6. Season the turkey and vegetables with dried thyme, sage, salt, and pepper. Stir to combine.
7. Once the squash is cooked, remove it from the oven and reduce the oven temperature to 350°F (175°C).
8. Fill half each acorn squash with the turkey and vegetable mixture, dividing it evenly among the halves.
9. Sprinkle the shredded mozzarella cheese over the top of each stuffed squash half.
10. Place the stuffed squash back in the oven and bake for 10-15 minutes until the cheese is melted and bubbly.
11. Garnish with fresh parsley before serving, if desired.

Nutrition Facts (per serving):
- Calories: 320
- Total Fat: 14g
- Saturated Fat: 4g
- Cholesterol: 80mg
- Sodium: 250mg
- Total Carbohydrates: 22g
- Dietary Fiber: 4g
- Sugars: 4g
- Protein: 27g

Mediterranean Chicken Skewers with Greek Salad
Cooking Time: 25 minutes
Serving: 4
Materials:
For Chicken Skewers:
- 1 lb (450g) boneless, skinless chicken breasts, cut into chunks
- One large red bell pepper, cut into chunks
- One large yellow bell pepper, cut into chunks
- One large red onion, cut into chunks
- One tablespoon olive oil
- Two cloves garlic, minced
- One teaspoon dried oregano
- One teaspoon dried thyme
- Salt and pepper to taste

- Wooden skewers, soaked in water for 30 minutes

For Greek Salad:

- Two large tomatoes, diced
- One cucumber, diced
- 1/2 red onion, thinly sliced
- 1/2 cup Kalamata olives, pitted
- 1/2 cup crumbled feta cheese
- Two tablespoons extra virgin olive oil
- One tablespoon red wine vinegar
- One teaspoon dried oregano
- Salt and pepper to taste

Steps:

1. **Preheat grill**: Preheat your grill to medium-high heat.
2. **Marinate chicken**: In a bowl, combine olive oil, minced garlic, dried oregano, dried thyme, salt, and pepper. Add chicken chunks to the bowl and toss until evenly coated. Let it marinate for at least 15 minutes.
3. **Prepare skewers**: Thread marinated chicken, bell peppers, and red onion alternately onto the soaked wooden skewers.
4. **Grill skewers**: Place the skewers on the preheated grill and cook for about 10-12 minutes, turning occasionally, until the chicken is cooked and the vegetables are tender and slightly charred.
5. **Make Greek Salad**: In a large bowl, combine diced tomatoes, diced cucumber, thinly sliced red onion, Kalamata olives, and crumbled feta cheese.
6. **Dress the salad**: In a small bowl, whisk together extra virgin olive oil, red wine vinegar, dried oregano, salt, and pepper. Pour the dressing over the salad and toss gently to combine.
7. **Serve**: Serve the Mediterranean Chicken Skewers hot off the grill with Greek Salad.

Nutrition Facts (per serving):

Note: Nutrition facts are approximate and may vary depending on the ingredients used.

- Calories: 320
- Total Fat: 16g
- Saturated Fat: 5g
- Cholesterol: 80mg
- Sodium: 560mg
- Total Carbohydrate: 13g
- Dietary Fiber: 4g

- Sugars: 7g
- Protein: 30g

Spaghetti Squash Pad Thai with Tofu

Cooking Time: 45 minutes
Serving: 4
Materials:
- One medium spaghetti squash
- 14 oz extra firm tofu, pressed and cubed
- One tablespoon vegetable oil
- Two cloves garlic, minced
- One red bell pepper, thinly sliced
- One carrot, julienned
- Three green onions, sliced
- 1 cup bean sprouts
- 1/4 cup chopped peanuts
- Lime wedges for serving
- Fresh cilantro for garnish
- Sesame seeds, for garnish

Pad Thai Sauce:
- Three tablespoons soy sauce
- Two tablespoons rice vinegar
- Two tablespoons brown sugar
- One tablespoon lime juice
- One tablespoon Sriracha sauce
- One teaspoon sesame oil

Steps:
1. **Prepare the Spaghetti Squash:** Preheat the oven to 375°F (190°C). Cut the spaghetti squash in half lengthwise and scoop out the seeds. Place the halves, cut side down, on a baking sheet lined with parchment paper. Bake for 30-40 minutes until the squash is tender and easily pierced with a fork. Once cooked, use a fork to scrape the squash into strands. Set aside.
2. **Prepare the Tofu:** Heat one tablespoon of vegetable oil in a large skillet over medium heat while the squash is baking. Add the cubed tofu and cook until golden brown on all sides, about 10-12 minutes. Remove tofu from the skillet and set aside.

3. **Make the Pad Thai Sauce:** In a small bowl, whisk together the soy sauce, rice vinegar, brown sugar, lime juice, Sriracha sauce, and sesame oil. Set aside.
4. **Cook the Vegetables:** In the same skillet used for tofu, add minced garlic, sliced red bell pepper, and julienned carrot. Sauté for 3-4 minutes until the vegetables are slightly softened.
5. **Combine Ingredients:** Add the cooked spaghetti squash strands, cooked tofu, sliced green onions, and bean sprouts to the skillet with the vegetables. Pour the Pad Thai sauce over the ingredients and toss everything together until well combined. Cook for an additional 2-3 minutes until heated through.
6. **Serve:** Divide the Spaghetti Squash Pad Thai among serving plates. Sprinkle with chopped peanuts and garnish with lime wedges, fresh cilantro, and sesame seeds. Serve immediately and enjoy!

Nutrition Facts (per serving):
- Calories: 280 kcal
- Total Fat: 15g
    - Saturated Fat: 2g
    - Trans Fat: 0g
- Cholesterol: 0mg
- Sodium: 780mg
- Total Carbohydrate: 26g
    - Dietary Fiber: 6g
    - Sugars: 11g
- Protein: 16g
- Vitamin D: 0%
- Calcium: 15%
- Iron: 20%
- Potassium: 660mg

Balsamic Glazed Pork Tenderloin with Roasted Brussels Sprouts
Cooking Time: 40 minutes
 Servings: 4
Materials:
- 1 lb pork tenderloin
- 1 lb Brussels sprouts, trimmed and halved
- Four tablespoons balsamic vinegar
- Two tablespoons honey
- Two cloves garlic, minced

- Two tablespoons olive oil
- Salt and pepper to taste
- Fresh rosemary sprigs for garnish

Steps:

1. Preheat your oven to 400°F (200°C).
2. Mix vinegar, honey, minced garlic, salt, and pepper. Set aside in a small bowl.
3. Place the trimmed and halved Brussels sprouts on a baking sheet. Drizzle with one tablespoon of olive oil and season with salt and pepper. Toss to coat evenly. Spread them out in a single layer.
4. Place the pork tenderloin on another baking sheet lined with parchment paper or aluminum foil. Season the pork with salt and pepper.
5. Brush the balsamic glaze mixture over the pork tenderloin and coat it evenly.
6. Place both the Brussels sprouts and the pork tenderloin in the preheated oven. Roast for about 25-30 minutes, or until the pork reaches an internal temperature of 145°F (63°C) and the Brussels sprouts are caramelized and tender.
7. Once cooked, remove the pork tenderloin from the oven and let it rest for 5 minutes before slicing.
8. Serve the sliced pork tenderloin alongside the roasted Brussels sprouts. Garnish with fresh rosemary sprigs if desired.

Nutrition Facts (per serving):

- Calories: 320
- Total Fat: 12g
- Saturated Fat: 3g
- Cholesterol: 80mg
- Sodium: 220mg
- Total Carbohydrate: 20g
- Dietary Fiber: 4g
- Sugars: 13g
- Protein: 32g

As you end the "Bariatric Meal Prep Cookbook," we hope you feel motivated and confident in taking charge of your health and well-being. Whether you have recently undergone bariatric surgery or are considering it in the future, please know that you are not alone on this journey.

Changing your diet and lifestyle can be challenging, but you can achieve your health goals and live your best life with the right tools, support, and mindset. Creating sustainable, lasting change takes time, patience, and dedication, but we assure you it is possible.

We encourage you to continue exploring new recipes, experimenting with different flavors, and discovering what works best for you and your body. Our cookbook is just the beginning of your journey to better health. Countless resources, including support groups, online communities, and professional guidance, are available to help you stay on track and motivated.

It's important to remember that progress is not always linear, and setbacks are a natural part of the process. However, what truly matters is staying committed to your health and moving forward, one step at a time. Small, consistent actions can lead to significant changes over time.

We hope the recipes, meal planning guides, and expert tips in this cookbook have been helpful resources for your health journey. Whether you want to lose weight, improve your overall health, or enjoy delicious and nutritious meals, we believe healthy eating can be both enjoyable and sustainable.

We want to thank you for allowing us to join your wellness journey. Your health and happiness are our top priority, and we are here to support you every step of the way. Here's to your long-term success!